D0726457

AUDIT IN MENTAL HEALTH SERVICES

Audit in Mental Health Services

A Guide to Carrying Out Clinical Audits for
Clinical Psychologists
Nurses
Occupational Therapists
Psychiatrists
Psychotherapists
Social Workers
and all health professionals involved in
mental health,
learning difficulties, and the elderly

Jenny Firth-Cozens

 LAWRENCE ERLBAUM ASSOCIATES, PUBLISHERS
Hove (UK)   Hillsdale (USA)

Lawrence Erlbaum Associates Ltd., Publishers
27 Palmeira Mansions
Church Road
Hove
East Sussex, BN3 2FA
U.K.

British Library Cataloguing in Publication Data
Firth-Cozens, Jenny
 Audit in Mental Health Services
 I. Title
 362.2028

ISBN 0-86377-311-7 (Pbk)

Printed and bound by BPCC Wheatons Ltd., Exeter

How To Use This Book

The book is written for individuals or teams who want to conduct meaningful audits—those which are designed to bring about an improvement in patient care.

In each chapter there are a number of exercises. These can be tackled individually, as a professional or multidisciplinary team, or in a workshop setting with larger numbers working in small groups.

Some of the exercises are designed to help you understand about audit—the benefits of the various methods, and so on—while others (marked with ♦) are more central to the audit programme you and your team will tackle: deciding on topics and methods, designing your outcomes, agreeing who should be influenced to bring about the change. The book stands without the exercises and so you may choose to ignore them, or to just do those which affect the stage of audit you are currently tackling.

Although the book is designed to get you started in audit, those who already have audits underway may simply want to skim the first few chapters and concentrate more on those concerned with methodology, outcomes, and change. Nevertheless, you may still want to return to earlier chapters when you want to develop your annual audit programme or to simply choose your next topic.

Jenny Firth-Cozens

AUTHOR'S BIOGRAPHY

Dr. Jenny Firth-Cozens, a Chartered Clinical and Occupational Psychologist, has been involved in the evaluation of clinical practice for a number of years, and was Regional Audit coordinator for the Yorkshire Regional Health Authority. As Principal Research Officer in Clinical Audit at the University of Leeds, she runs courses and workshops on medical and clinical audit for various professional groups and for multidisciplinary teams. In her consultancy practice she works with local audit committees on the facilitation of audit, and with health service and community teams on strategic issues, evaluation, and team development

ACKNOWLEDGEMENTS

My thanks go to Dr. Adrian Bull, Consultant in Public Health at Eastbourne DHA who worked with me on introducing audit in the Yorkshire region. And thanks also to the doctors and other health professionals who took part in the workshops which formed the basis for this book.

Contents

CHAPTER ONE

Introduction

A BRIEF HISTORY OF CLINICAL AUDIT[1]

Clinical audit is a way of systematically reviewing and improving the quality of care we give to patients. Such audits are not new. Many readers will be able to think of occasions in the past when they have gathered data to understand better what is going on in their clinic, and have often brought about change as a result. In the late 1980s some of these activities were funded by Regional Health Authorities (RHAs) with the express purpose of encouraging clinical audits to be conducted by all health professionals, sometimes working in a multidisciplinary way (e.g. a day hospital or a community team), sometimes with a single professional group.

A change in emphasis came about with the publication of the 1989 White Paper, Working for Patients, which introduced major innovations in health care provision through contracting, resource management and medical audit. The introduction of medical audit—audit by medical groups—was facilitated by large sums of ring-fenced Department of Health (DoH) money, distributed by RHAs to District Audit Committees, usually consisting of a group of consultants representing most specialties, but

---

[1]Many of you will be aware of what has happened in the National Health Service to formalise this process into a requirement, and what some of the routes for its funding have been. This section is for those who want to remind themselves of what the key steps have been in its history.

occasionally including a manager or clinical psychologist or nurse. One or two trusts chose to make their audit committee representative of all health professionals, establishing true clinical audit from the outset.

Initially, the funding was often used for buying computer systems. It was quickly discovered, however, that these frequently did not deliver what was hoped for in terms of being easy to use and adaptable, and that audits were still often done just as well without them. Now, increasingly, the money is being used to pay for medical audit coordinators (or officers, or assistants, or a host of other names) who help to organise audit activity, to conduct audits with specialist teams, and sometimes to educate others in audit methods (Firth-Cozens & Venning, 1991).

Although there has been some money delivered down a nursing route for clinical audit by nurses and professionals allied to medicine (PAMs), this is very small compared to the medical audit money and few, if any, staff have been taken on as clinical audit coordinators in the same way that has happened with medical audit. As the need to consider all the elements that make up the process and outcome of care become appreciated, clinical audit will develop out of medical audit. In particular, as audit and quality become increasingly a part of the commissioning debate—as the specification of both systems and outcomes are reflected within contracts between purchasers and providers—then clinical rather than medical audit becomes not just desirable, but inevitable.

The Benefits of Multidisciplinary Audits

In mental health the trend towards multidisciplinary teams has encouraged audit to continue in its original form. It is generally agreed that the different professional contributions to inpatient and outpatient care and especially to community mental health care are often difficult to distinguish. Therefore the quality of care needs to be audited by all those concerned in its delivery, and the need for a multidisciplinary approach has also been encouraged by the Royal College of Psychiatrists.

There is no doubt that it can be difficult to cross rigid professional boundaries and begin to question, as a team, what is best for patients rather than shoring up defences to awkward questions. But it is undoubtedly better for the patient that care really does represent a unified package designed for quality. Most teams eventually agree that it is better for them too. Teams whose membership is extremely similar never do as well as those which recognise and enjoy their diversity—whether this is of individual traits or of professional know-how. Audit is an excellent way to develop the multidisciplinary team since it allows a variety of different tasks and roles and so can use a diversity of skills.

DEFINITIONS OF CLINICAL AUDIT

Medical audit was defined by the DoH in Working Paper 6 as:

> ... a systematic, critical analysis of the quality of medical care, including the procedures used for diagnosis and treatment, resources and the resulting outcome and quality of life for the patient.

In addition to this definition, many of the principal non-medical professional groups who are involved in mental health care services—nurses, clinical psychologists, speech therapists, and occupational therapists—have put forward their own definitions of clinical audit. For example, the NHS Management Executive's paper (NHSME, 1991), "Framework of Audit for Nursing Services" described it in this way:

> Nursing Audit is part of the cycle of Quality Assurance. It incorporates the systematic and critical analysis by nurses, midwives and health visitors, in conjunction with other staff, of the planning, delivery and evaluation of nursing and midwifery care, in terms of their use of resources and the outcomes for patients/clients, and introduces appropriate change in response to that analysis.

The College of Occupational Therapy (quoted in Merrall et al., 1991) describe audit as:

> A methodical review or investigation of resources and activities both clinically and managerially, a means of quality promotion whereby a group of peers within one discipline decides criteria of good performance and then audits their records to find the level of competence.

The College of Speech and Language Therapists (1991) stated that clincial audit is:

> ... the formal mechanism set up to evaluate the ability of the individual and or service to adhere to the quality standards as described. Clinical audit is the evaluation of clinical outcomes...achieved through the audit of the actual outcome of a therapeutic intervention against the expected outcomes as hypothesised at the outset of the intervention.

Clinical psychologists have not defined audit formally, but many clinical psychology services have regularly audited their outcomes for the last few years (Parry, 1992).

Most medical specialties have accepted the Working Party 6 definitions, but the Royal College of Psychiatrists has appreciated the obvious need for audit to be a multidisciplinary activity rather than one carved out by separate professional groups, and has recommended the term "clinical audit" rather than "medical audit". In fact, clinical audit is now seen as the way forward by the DoH.

Exercise 1.1: Common and Individual Elements

> As a group, whether from your own profession or one consisting of the various professions with whom you work, consider these definitions and write down the elements that most of them have in common, and those that seem to be particular to one profession.

Common Factors   *Individual Factors*

Comment: Some of the factors common to all the definitions are:

1. The audit will be systematic, methodical, and analytical. This implies that the question it asks will be addressed scientifically, although not in the way that research might address it (see p.9 on the differences between audit and research).

2. Its emphasis will be on quality of care, whether this is looking at the process or procedures leading up to treatment, the treatment itself, or the outcome. In addition, two of the definitions mention resources, implying that it might look at the cost-effectiveness of treatments or procedures.

3. Two of the definitions mention outlining of standards or criteria against which to conduct the audit and compare your results with those you might expect from the standards you have set. This was left out of the original definition of medical audit, with the result that doctors were often confused by what was expected of them, and many regarded the simple case discussion that had always taken place as sufficient for audit. Increasingly, the various professional associations and colleges are emphasising the importance of setting standards in order to conduct audits.

There are other specific points within the definitions worth commenting on. For example, the occupational therapy definition includes the possibility of an audit of "activities". This was very much the type of audit that Kohner data were used for and its usefulness in terms of improving patient care is very doubtful. Most people would agree that good **outcomes** in terms of patient care are much more important than any level of activity, and so the emphasis has generally shifted away from this type of audit.

The speech therapy definition refers to "levels of competence", which has not appeared elsewhere and might well raise qualms in most health workers. It is certainly not a prime aim of audit, medical or clinical, that individual levels of competence will be assessed. The introduction of medical audit has very much emphasised that only group data will be available to anyone outside the specialty group. Nevertheless, in reality it is clear that individual competence may at some point become an issue; for example, to fund-holding general practitioners who may make assessments of the care given to their patients by individuals to whom they are referred.

A point which appears only in the occupational therapist definition, is that **audits will be conducted by your peers**. Although this was not part of the medical audit definition, it has been seen as vitally important. When audit was first introduced, evaluation by one's peers was regarded as sacrosanct with some consultants even excluding junior doctors and audit officers from meetings. Certainly other professional groups were only occasionally included. But there is no doubt that the definition of one's "peers" is changing and becoming broader as audit is seen as increasingly useful and the fears about what it might reveal are lessening.

Your "peers" may be:

* Those within your professional department (e.g. clinical psychology).
* Those within a specialty (e.g. psychiatry/geriatric medicine).
* Those within a multidisciplinary team (e.g. an alcohol and drug unit, or a day hospital).
* Those involved in the audit (e.g. the audit officer, the appointment clerk, even the general manager—whoever is appropriate, see Chapter 2, p.12).

In small specialties, such as child and adolescent psychiatry, psychiatrists meet regionally to conduct audits. Within psychotherapy, those interested meet nationally and have the Service Evaluation Group. However, with the advent of trusts this will become less appropriate and the question "Who are my peers?" is much more likely to be answered within your clinical group. There is still an important place, however, for audit to be discussed and developed within your professional group, so that more specialised measures and methods can be developed.

Finally, only the nursing definition mentions "change in response to the analysis". **Change** in terms of improvements in patient care is what audit is all about. We need to keep this primary goal very firmly in mind throughout our audit activity if it is to remain meaningful and even enjoyable.

VIEWS ABOUT AUDIT

Most of you will have some idea of what is involved in clinical audit. Some will have taken part in audits with a variety of levels of sophistication. Many of you will hold views about its more formalised introduction, and some of these opinions will be strongly for or against. Before going any further, it is worthwhile airing these views.

EXERCISE 1.2: Views about Audit

> Work in small groups to discuss the pros and cons of clinical audit.
> List these under the headings of *Benefits* and *Disadvantages* and
> then share them in a plenary.

Benefits of Audit   *Disadvantages of Audit*

Comment: You may well have found that the list of advantages is just as long as the list of disadvantages. That is certainly what happened in workshops I ran with mixed groups of consultants in the early days of clinical audit (Bull & Firth-Cozens, 1991). Table 1.1 shows a summary of consultants' views at that time.

Dealing with Difficulties

Whatever the problems raised in Exercise 2, chances are that you mentioned the difficulties of finding time, of confidentiality or management intrusion, and of computing. You may have said that you cannot look at what are really research questions by conducting audits. It is useful to discuss these points before continuing, though it is likely that they will remain issues to address as circumstances change, and as your use of audit increases. If none of them were problems for you, then move on to the next section.

TABLE 1.1
Benefits and Disadvantages of Audit

Benefits	Disadvantages
Improved patient care	Time
Teaching/education	Clinical freedom
Research	Staff resistance/inertia
Brings together various disciplines	?Leaving gaps (cannot audit everything)
Ring-fenced money	Confidentiality
More attention will be paid	"Big Brother"
Audit will direct us towards research areas	No training/facilities
Job satisfaction	Judging by numbers
Political } Useful information provided Financial	Tedious Adminstrative only
Improved medical practice	Difficulties in assessing outcome
Improved efficiency in hospital	Poor data—small numbers
Setting standards—medico-legal help	Cost-limiting exercise
Comparisons with peers	Implementing outcomes—will managers
Identification of problems	want to know that more money is needed?
Overlap with resource management	Poor IT (including personnel)
Rationalisation of protocols	Implications for contracting
Working cross-speciality	Will it lead to uniformity of practice?
Teamwork should improve	Junior doctors are only here 6 months— causing low satisfaction
	Colleagues not collecting data
	Small specialties
	Rare illness may be overlooked

From Bull and Firth-Cozens (1991).

Finding Time

Many health professionals argue that the time taken up in audit could be better spent caring for patients. Certainly, audit will become a regular part of your working week, but it is argued—and individual audits confirm this—that savings on time can be achieved through audit. Although it is too early to say whether this will represent an overall saving, if your audits provide only one opportunity to save time each year, this will be cumulative. The mere discussion with colleagues about the best way to tackle something often results in one or two individuals realising that there are alternatives which might save time, and even improve patient care as well.

In addition, most people agree that audit should also be educational, especially when linked to supervision, and as such it should be a particularly efficient and effective way of continuing professional education.

In any case, attention to the standards of our care and the outcomes we are achieving is unarguably essential for any professional group, especially those responsible for the safety or the lives of others.

What we need to ask is not whether we have time for audit, but whether it makes any sense at all to be putting so much effort into care without actually examining what we do and the way we do it. We need to know if this is in the best interests of our patients, and even whether it is making any real contribution to their care. All good work practice requires time for reflection, and audit provides a structured way of doing that on a regular basis.

Do You Need Computer Systems?

In the early days of clinical audit, many groups paid vast amounts of money to install computers which had special audit software. Their audit time went largely into trying to understand the system and to fit it to their needs, and this often met with failure and disillusionment about audit. Groups that progressed with audit activity and could actually report useful change as a result were frequently those without computers, or with small inexpensive personal computers with simple software not specifically designed for audit.

It's true that if you are seeing large numbers of patients, or if you will want to separate out groups of patients (e.g. those of a certain age, or a certain diagnosis, or being offered a particular therapy), then it is much easier to have a personal computer (PC) and simple statistical software. Some of those found useful are described in Chapter 6.

"Audit is Just a Management Tool"

There is no doubt that many general managers are becoming aware of the importance of audit, both as a way of increasing efficiency and as a way of meeting and measuring the quality demands of purchasers. There is still a dearth of good useful information in the health service, and audit, being local, relevant, and narrowly focused on a particular problem or procedure should, if it is done well, provide very useful information to managers as well as to clinicians.

This doesn't mean that audit has a "Big Brother" element aimed at singling out the person whose work is below standard. Although it may well have the capability of doing this, most managers, general practitioners, and even the cleaner on the ward are able to tell you that a particular doctor or therapist is not up to scratch. You probably know surgeons you would trust and those you would rather avoid; or you could find this information fairly easily if you tried. Audit should not be made responsible for what has always been common knowledge.

In terms of managers using audit to reduce costs, this is possible, but it is equally likely that many audits will also reveal the need for extra expenditure. It is important that this is taken into account if managers want to see audit really doing its job and bringing about improvements.

The only foreseeable problem in this area could be for those who do not set up satisfactory audit mechanisms in trusts. There is then the likelihood that audits of their practice will be externally developed by purchasers. Many people involved in audit nationally see this as a realistic reason to produce good in-house audit systems.

Audit and Research

In the majority of audits there will no confusion over what is audit and what is research. In outcome audits, however—looking at the effectiveness of some aspect of care—there may be some staff who raise the issue that this can only be considered with a research design. But audit is not research: It has a very different purpose. Although the purpose of audit is to evaluate how closely our own practice is to best practice, research aims to establish what that best practice actually is. So, if research tells you that 70 per cent of depressed patients are significantly improved by a particular combination of imipramine and cognitive-behavioural therapy, then your audit might indicate that your own depressed patients, given that treatment, are improving at that rate.

The data you collect should be able to tell you why you are exceeding that standard of practice or not meeting it. For example, by measuring people's depression at admission, using the same inventory as the original outcome research, you should be able to see if your patients are more severely depressed than theirs were, or if they had longer or shorter time for therapy, and so on. Such questions are discussed in detail in Chapters 4 to 6.

Research is designed in such a way to ensure that it can be replicated and that its results apply to other similar groups. Audit, on the other hand, is specific and local to your own particular patient group. It should not be used to compare your group with those in other districts or other hospitals, because it hasn't taken all the precautions of sampling which is necessary in research. Some people regard audit as inadequate for this reason, but in fact it may be far more helpful to conduct audit with your own idiosyncratic but heterogeneous patient group than simply to rely on the research findings from a sample rare in its homogeneity. Most mental health outcome research is enormously lengthy and expensive, and many of the criticisms of it centre on the fact that, in the end, both its clients and its manualised treatments and therapies bear little relation to real clinical practice (Parry, 1992). Nevertheless, using the results as a standard by which to compare your practice does give you a useful baseline to consider how well you are doing.

Other important distinctions between audit and research are, for example, that the reporting of research findings takes place in the public arena, whereas with audit only grouped data (not identifying patient or clinician) are made available, and then only to the unit's audit committee. As purchasers play an increasing role in requesting audits, they will, of course have access to results and the division between public and internal reporting will become more blurred. In research it should be possible to reproduce your results again and again; in audit it would be a very poor first audit if it hadn't brought about change, and so reproducing your results is seen as undesirable. Finally, politics is not seen as part of research, but it is usually recognised as inevitable in some audits; for example, if you want to make a case to continue a particular service you are increasingly going to have to provide good audit data to back up your argument.

Although the distinctions between audit and research seem clear enough, in practice there is something of an overlap, particularly in mental health care. For example, while much can be learned by additive data only, more can occasionally be gained by using appropriate simple statistical tests, such as correlations. In fact, given a good audit design there is no reason why you shouldn't publish audits if you want. The British Medical Association journal, *Quality in Health Care,* exists both as a vehicle for publishing actual audits, and for more academic and research papers about quality, measurement, and outcome.

CHAPTER TWO

The Audit Meeting

THE PURPOSE OF THE AUDIT MEETING

The audit meeting should let the group:

* Choose an audit topic.
* Discuss and record what constitutes good care.
* Design an audit.
* Discuss raw data.
* Agree the audit report.
* Decide what changes should be made.

Of course this will not all take place within the same meeting; on the other hand, you may consider aspects of two or more ongoing audits within one meeting.

TIME TO MEET

Most doctors meet for one session a month to design and discuss their audits. This is usually sufficient time for these tasks, although it presupposes that data collection takes place between these meetings. Where data collection is retrospective (see Chapter 4, p.31), this will entail a task in itself, usually for one individual, such as a trainee, junior doctor or audit officer. However, where it is prospective, perhaps using a single data sheet, this will be done by all levels of the team on whichever patients they see who fall within the parameters of the audit.

Other professional groups don't always have the benefit of half a day a month carved out of their time especially for audit. Instead they may try to meet weekly in a lunch-hour or tacked on to the end of a department meeting, for example. This is rarely enough time to go into all the issues of design—agreeing on a topic, choosing a method, setting standards, etc.—and these tasks are better done in a half day setting, or two sessions, if standards are to be developed by the team itself. In some hospitals, everyone has a session a month for audit on the basis of a rolling half day, and this is ideal for cross-specialty or multidisciplinary work.

However you decide to allocate your time for audit, remember that the usefulness of the results will only be in proportion to the quality of the initial design. It really is worthwhile putting most of your efforts into this initial phase even if it means that the audit seems slow in getting off the ground.

THE ORGANISATION OF THE MEETING

Whether you are auditing within your professional group or in a multidisciplinary team, or in a regional group (e.g. where professional numbers are very small), you should appoint one person to be responsible for organising the meetings and circulating any action plans that arise from them. This isn't a job for the newest, youngest member, but for someone who has enough status and assertiveness to deal with some inevitable resistance and cynicism that come with change and with the difficulties of evaluation. Initially, it may be best if this person also chairs the meetings, but once the audit process is underway, it's more useful to rotate this position so that everyone has an equal chance to be involved.

It may seem a small point, but providing coffee and biscuits (if not lunch) makes audit meetings more attractive. If you have audit funds, spend some on "hospitality".

Several medical colleges require participants to sign in on their attendance at audit meetings for the purpose of getting training recognition. Even when this is not necessary, it is a good idea to record the names of all the attenders so that the cost of audits can be estimated for contracting purposes.

WHO SHOULD BE INVOLVED?

There is a golden rule in audit. It says: **You can never audit anyone else's practice** Although you can easily collect data on what other people are doing in terms of audit, you can't then make them change their practice if this is shown necessary from the data. We know, from research in occupational psychology, that people are much more amenable to change if they are involved from the beginning. Because of this, it's a good idea to talk with everyone you think might be necessary right from the design stage. For example, if you decide to look at waiting times for outpatients, you will need to involve the appointments clerk and possibly the ambulance drivers' manager as well.

But it's not always possible to know in advance just who is going to be necessary. If you find, as a result of your audit, that other groups should be brought in, then do that when you set new parameters and then re-audit the topics with them. (Involvement of others will be looked at in more detail in Chapter 7.)

Ideally, an audit officer should also attend your meetings, but they tend to be too thin on the ground to do that for every specialty. Do at least let them know what you're doing, however, and invite them to attend when a new audit is being designed. Their experience in this should be very valuable.

Finally (and I appreciate the irony of the word used here), you might consider having a patient/user/client/carer as a member of your audit group—perhaps someone co-opted as appropriate to help in the design of a specific audit. This has only happened in one or two places but it seems a very good idea: Patient views on what is a good outcome might be different to those who care for them. Of course, confidentiality would mean they could not attend meetings where raw data are discussed.

◆ Exercise 2.1: Defining Your Audit Group

(a) Will you have a group limited to your profession, or a multidisciplinary group, or both?

(b) Decide now who will be the core members of your audit group.

(c) Who will be the leader, responsible for pushing the audit along, negotiating with managers and the chair of the local audit committee, and so on?

(d) Who will chair your meetings?

THE PAPERWORK OF AUDIT

The Audit Meeting Record

Figures 2.1 and 2.2 show two examples of the record of an audit meeting, developed in general hospitals. They include obvious details, such as the date and the names of those present and apologies for absence, as well as the title of the audit. The centre sections include details of what has been decided in terms of design and responsibilities, which is applicable in the initial stages of an audit. The last sections include details of changes agreed as a result of the audit data and the meeting, who needs to be informed, what action will be taken, and by whom. How you design your own record sheet will depend on your needs. It would be worth spending a few minutes to think about whether those illustrated here are sufficient, or what might make them better for you.

Ideally, the record sheets will be confidential to your group. However, with the blurring of boundaries between managers and clinicians that has come about, this may not always be the case. Certainly some medical colleges require evidence of adequate attendance in order to grant accreditation for training posts, and this is likely to occur with other professional groups as well. I can imagine that managers who view audit as an essential part of all professionals' activity (e.g. those who provide a rolling half day for everyone) would want to know they had access to the records of attendance if they wanted them.

Whether or not they are involved in the audit, the audit officer should receive a copy so that she or he is of aware what audits are happening and may, for example, be able to put you in touch with other groups in the region undertaking similar audits. They might even know where there might be funds available to carry this out.

The Data Sheets from Audits

Many of your meetings will be considering **raw data** from completed audits, and these might allow identification of individual professionals or of patients. This level of data is currently seen as being for the eyes of the audit group alone, and so most groups do not keep it once it has been considered and aggregated. Remember that the Data Protection Act (1984) allows patients access to data held on computers and word processors, while the Access to Health Records Act (1990) allows access to written records.

The **aggregated data**—showing means and percentages, for example—**and its accompanying report** become the public face of audit for your multidisciplinary team or your professional group. For this reason there must be no reference to individual professionals or patients.

CLINICAL AUDIT: DEPARTMENT/DIRECTORATE NOTES

This form is to help Departments/Directorates to record each of their medical audit meetings and to help the DMAC to build up a picture of audit activity across the District.

Directorate/Department _____

Audit Meeting Date _____

Meeting began _____ am/pm   ended _____ am/pm

Present_____   Absent _____

_____   _____

_____   _____

1.Topic   _____

    _____

    Action Plans   _____

    _____

    Review Date _____
    Action Coordinator   _____

2.Topic   _____

    _____

    Action Plans   _____

    _____

    Review Date _____
    Action Coordinator   _____

3.Topic   _____

    _____

    Action Plans   _____

    _____

    Review Date _____
    Action Coordinator   _____

4.Topic   _____

    _____

    Action Plans   _____

    _____

    Review Date _____
    Action Coordinator   _____

5.Topic   _____

    _____

    Action Plans   _____

    _____

    Review Date _____
    Action Coordinator   _____

Date of next meeting   _____

Signed   _____

(Lead Consultant)

Copy to: District Medical Audit Committee Chair

FIG. 2.1. Audit Meeting Record.

MINUTES OF MEDICAL AUDIT MEETING

AUDIT GROUP   _____

DATE OF MEETING   _____

VENUE   _____

PRESENT AT MEETING

NAME   DESIGNATION   SPECIALTY

TO BE RETAINED BY AUDIT GROUP

- -

MINUTES OF MEDICAL AUDIT MEETING

AUDIT GROUP   _____

DATE OF MEETING   _____

VENUE   _____

TOPICS DISCUSSED:

CONCLUSIONS ARISING OUT OF MEETING:

PROPOSALS FOR CHANGE/ACTION

DATE AND VENUE OF NEXT MEETING:
1 copy to be retained by Audit Group; 1 copy to Medical Audit Officer

---

FIG. 2.2. Audit Meeting Record.

Depending on how audit is organised in your district or trust—that is, whether it is handled by a medical audit committee or if there is a clinical audit committee representing all professionals—these aggregated results will be made available to the chair of the audit committee, or to the appropriate service manager if you are non-medical and not working in a multidisciplinary way.

The Unit Audit Report

This is usually compiled by the audit officers and chair of the local audit committee. It is a summary of audit activity in the unit or trust and the findings and changes which have come about. Eventually, it will be evidence that you have fulfilled contractual obligations with purchasers. Table 2.1 summarises the paperwork required for audit.

TABLE 2.1
The Paperwork of Audit

Audit meeting record	Records the topic, what's agreed, action to be taken and by whom, and attendance. Possible access by colleges and managers if time has been given to attend audit meetings.
Raw data	Non-aggregated. Not kept on computer or elsewhere.
Audit reports with aggregated data	Public documents for chair of district/trust audit committee, and possibly management.
Unit/trust audit report	Summarises all the audit activities and changes brought about, for the benefit of senior managers and purchasers.

Confidentiality

All this raises questions about how much access will actually be given to audit records and reports, both in terms of what future purchasers might demand and in terms of litigation. Basically, the answer is that we don't know. Although there is a defence in litigation that disclosure is not in the public interest, this has not yet been tested in any court, and it is quite likely that the records from individual clinicians or groups could be used. Setting out local confidentiality guidelines is essential.

There is also a positive side to audit and litigation. It might be possible that, in the process of deciding local practice in terms of standards and criteria of care, you are able to point out local limitations. Provided you are meeting the standards and criteria set within those limitations, then this may be a defence which would be considered by a court. Again, however, as there has been no such case, no one can be sure.

♦ Exercise 2.2: Data and Confidentiality

(a) Decide on the design of an audit meeting record and the information it will regularly include.

(b) Discuss and agree how you will deal with confidentiality in terms of all the documentation and data of your audit group.

CHAPTER THREE

Choosing a Topic

INTRODUCTION

The NHS has collected data in staggering quantities ever since its inception. Anyone who has been subject to completing Kohner forms or any other type of activity audit is probably more than a little jaundiced against collecting even more data. The main problem with such exercises is that the staff do not own the data in any way and that there is usually no feedback or changes made for the benefits of patients (at least none that were apparent) as a result of what the data revealed.

Clinical audit is very different. It is initiated by you to answer questions in which you are interested, ones that you actually care about. The data you collect is your data, and the changes you make as a result of what the audit reveals are initiated by you. It is important to keep this in mind when you are choosing topics: choose those which are of interest or importance to yourself and/or to as many individuals within your team as possible. In addition, there are ways of classifying topics which will help you to narrow down the choice and to make your audits cover all aspects of patient care.

STRUCTURE, PROCESS, AND OUTCOME

Various systems have been proposed for choosing an area in which to audit care, most of them under the overarching title of "quality". Medical or clinical audit is a part of the more general search for quality, and so a number of topics are bound to overlap. The easiest way to see the relation between the two is through Donabedian's (1964) classification of topic areas. He divided quality investigations into the following:

Structure: The suitability of waiting rooms, appointment systems, equipment, staffing levels, of the usability and contents of patients' notes, and so on.

Process: The appropriateness of tests and procedures used, communication between professionals and patients or their relatives, continuity of who sees a patient on different occasions, and so on.

Outcome: The effectiveness and efficiency of treatment, such as clinical outcomes and cost-efficiency, but also quality of life and patient satisfaction.

In terms of the relationship between quality and audit within a hospital or community service, managers will be more responsible for the structure or quality end of the classification, while clinicians and other health professionals will be more responsible for the outcome end. As audit becomes increasingly defined within contracts, managers' interest is bound to grow in terms of understanding outcome results and requesting certain audits to be completed.

Of course, the divisions are not precise. Many of the aspects of process will depend on others generally seen as structure. For example, you may not be carrying out necessary procedures (process) because of inadequate or non-existent equipment (structure). Having appropriate levels of staff as a whole is usually seen as structure, but it may be a standard set in order to achieve a particular outcome. For example, first-year clinical psychology trainees may have their patients restricted in terms of severity; or a minimum grade of anaesthetist may be set as a criterion of care to ensure minimum complications in ECT.

Process and outcome also overlap: in many **chronic conditions** there may be no overall outcome, and so one aspect of process may be a regular check of symptom levels. In this case, process becomes a series of mini-outcomes.

In terms of using this structure to help you choose an audit topic, I would recommend that groups or individuals just beginning to audit should first choose a structure topic, and then one concerning process, before going on to tackle outcome.

An early emphasis on structure is useful for the following reasons:

1. It is relatively simple to audit and to get useful results and so it is a good way of getting your audit mechanisms started: holding

regular meetings, assigning tasks, ensuring accurate review, and generally appreciating what's involved in the process of doing audit.

2. The results will be within the immediate interests of management. Unless it is an audit which simply requires more money rather than other forms of change, this will let managers know that funding and encouraging your audit activity is particularly worthwhile. Relationships with managers is discussed more fully in Chapter 7, p.78.

3. Auditing structural aspects of care is by far the least threatening area for staff involved. There is no point pretending that audit doesn't have its threatening side—none of us likes being evaluated—and so to choose a topic which evaluates less intrinsic aspects of our care is easier to accept.

Of course, those readers who have already been auditing for some time will probably want to dive into the more difficult areas of process and outcome audits, and these will certainly become increasingly important as contracting becomes more sophisticated.

Comment: Another way of subdividing by quality areas uses a classification of topics based on those described some years ago in the *British Medical Journal* by Maxwell (1984).

QUALITY AREAS

According to this classification, services should have:

Equity: Everyone should have equal services in terms of the other quality areas; for example, there should be equity of access, or communication, or treatment delivery. An audit question in this category might ask whether information booklets are provided in all the locally used languages.

Access: Everyone should have sufficiently prompt access to the appropriate level of services; for example, people should not have to wait too long, or travel too far. They should see the right grade of professional, and so on. The category might include Patient Charter questions about the waiting list or the time taken to wait in outpatients; or it might audit a standard about what should be done to ensure an adequate assessment.

Acceptability and Responsiveness: The care offered, and the way it is offered, should be acceptable to the patient and accurately responsive to his or her needs. This is the one topic area where the patient's views are essential; they would be useful in all the other areas, but only the patients or their relatives can say if the service was acceptable or not.

Appropriateness: The treatments offered to the patients should only be carried out in circumstances where they are indicated; for example, are people being offered group therapy only where that is what will suit them best? Are their medication levels appropriate. Are appropriate tests being carried out; for example, psycho-neurological assessments, or thyroid function tests?

Communication: Any aspects of communication can be audited; for example, between staff and patient or patient's relatives as well as between professionals. So you might ask, are the notes made sufficient for another member of the team to understand what has been happening? Is the discharge letter adequate for the general practitioner to follow on the treatment? Is there access to interpreters, to people who can sign, and so on?

Continuity: Is the same staff member seeing the patient or carer regularly, or are there discontinuities? Where there are discontinuities—for example in a busy outpatients or drop-in centre—are the same principles of care being applied and are the notes sufficiently clear on this?

Effectiveness: This area focuses on outcomes and asks if the care or treatment offered is as effective as research or guidelines say it should be. This is the area which is central to the agenda of the next few years; it is also the most difficult. It is very important here, more than anywhere else, that audit and research are not confused. (See 1.3.4) Audit can't tell you whether treatment A is more effective than treatment B—only research can do that—but it can tell you whether you or your group's practice is as effective as research says it should be.

Efficiency: This is concerned with questions about whether as much is being achieved with the resources available to you as is possible? For example, research shows that on average there is minimal symptom improvement after 26 sessions of psychotherapy. You could therefore audit the reasons why longer therapy is chosen for some patients and then set criteria for choosing longer therapy in the future.

DEVELOPING AN AUDIT PROGRAMME

Exercise 3.1 will enable you to consider possible topics within your practice, with a view to beginning to map out a future audit program for your service. It will be worth photo-copying your prepared page onto at least A3 paper, so that you can use it over and over. Don't expect to complete it quickly. Choosing topics to audit can easily take up a whole audit session. Although the table you create in the exercise will be refined further, it will form the basis of your programme, and so the time spent will be well worth it.

♦ EXERCISE 3.1: Preparing Your Audit Programme

Prepare a page with a four column grid and plenty of space, and insert the following three headings: Structure, Process, and Outcome. Down the left-hand column, list the Quality Areas that have been outlined on pages 21/2. Under each of the three headings and in the appropriate boxes, list the audit topics within your field, preferably in the form of a question.

Compare your table with Table 3.1 on page 24. There will be slight variations in classification, and you are bound to have different topics, but that is fine: the purpose of the exercise is for you to generate topics, rather than to agree entirely with a particular classification.

Further guidelines for choosing relevant topics follow, and Exercise 3.2 will allow you to refine these by adding more practical concerns to your topic areas.

	Structure	Process	Outcome
Equity			
Access			
etc.			

TABLE 3.1

	Structure	Process	Outcome
Equity and access	Availability of psychotherapy service. Day hospital relief for carers. Standards set for level of community staff. Conditions in community homes	Minority languages catered for in terms of interpreters, bilingual professional. Waiting times for assessment, outpatients. Patients' Charter	Does DNA rate reduce when interpreters available?
Acceptability and responsiveness	Patient satisfaction with wards, community homes, access to senior staff. Are the services offered reflecting patient needs?	Patient and carer's satisfaction with communication, responsiveness to needs, frequency of appointments, etc.	Was outcome acceptable in terms of quality of life, satisfaction, family dynamics, etc?
Appropriateness	Do we have appropriately trained staff for the patients we see? Survey of security arrangement of rooms used by psychiatrists to assess emergency referrals. Conditions of consulting rooms	Are our physical investigations appropriate? Are we giving CBT, psychotherapy, OT, play therapy, group therapy, etc., when appropriate? Are particular patient groups seeing appropriate levels and types of professional? Are patients receiving appropriate psychometric testing? OT and nursing assessment.	Does drop-out reduce when appropriate assessments are conducted?
Communication	Are our notes maintained in an acceptable manner? Do we have easy access to information for patients? Are our confidentiality procedures adequate?	Do letters to GPs have sufficient information? Are our communications to each member of the team acceptable? Do we make it clear to patients' relatives the treatment options that are possible/available?	Is outcome communicated sufficiently well to patients/relatives, GPs and other community staff?
Continuity	Where continuity of care is not possible, are notes maintained to ensure similar care?	Do patients have continuity of care from one person where that is called for? Followup of patients referred from general hospital to addiction unit.	Is there continuity in aftercare? Respite care.
Effectiveness	Are wards/hostels, etc. sufficiently clean?	Is alcohol/drug dependency "absent" at each appointment? Are we maintaining patient compliance in drug therapy? Are community patients competent in necessary life skills? Is our proportion of bedsores meeting national standards?	Are our outcomes in short-term therapy as good as they should be? What are our long-term outcomes for substance abuse, truancy, carers' health, marital discord, sexual abuse, independence, etc? Is our relapse/readmission rate meeting our standards?
Efficiency	Procedure for reducing non-attendance is being followed.	Are tests, procedures, seclusions, drugs, therapies given only when indicated? Time spent travelling.	Is the length of therapy no longer than is necessary according to research?

CHOOSING A TOPIC THAT MATTERS

Audits should be on topics which matter to you, your team, your patients, and your community. Above all, they should be meaningful to you. This is what gives the findings a breath of fresh air compared with the usual data collections.

This is reflected in the final points to consider when choosing a topic area. The audit should particularly concern itself with areas that are:

High Risk
Expensive
Very Common
Very Rare
Of Local Concern

In the light of the remarks above, you should also take into account:

The Interest of You and Your Team
The Avoidance of a Problem or Condition
The Political Expediency of an Area
Requests from Purchasers

For example, if you are noticing (as many services are) that you have an increasing number of women patients who are referred for various symptoms relating to being sexually abused as children, you might want to audit aspects of your service to them. This would be because most research shows their treatment is **expensive**, in terms of often being very long-term; increasingly **common** (although it seems it was there but previously hidden under other diagnoses or within social services); and of **local concern**, especially to GPs. If your service is within an area where there are large ethnic minorities, it would also be important in terms of local concern to tackle aspects of your service to them.

If you find yourself constantly hunting through patients' notes for bits of information that are particularly important to you, then an audit which tackles the standards of note-keeping is a good idea in terms of being a **common problem and expensive** in terms of time lost.

Again, a useful audit in terms of high risk would be to followup parasuicides from A&E to find out where they go next. If guidelines to what should happen have been formulated as criteria, then these criteria could be audited. A team might decide that some aspects of bedsore prevention in the elderly, or hip fractures on wards are **common enough** and preventable enough to be audited.

Rare conditions are hardly ever subject to agreed protocols of care, and so it may be worth tackling these. It is expensive in terms of time to design audits about conditions which present so infrequently, but very inexpensive from then on, since data collection will be spasmodic.

Finally, you may wish to audit something in order to make a point about **the usefulness of your service or the need for extra funding** for one aspect of it. Although politics is not regarded as being correct within research, provided that your data is accurate and your audit well designed, then there is no reason to think that politics should not be a part of audit. Managers are still fairly bereft of good relevant information, so will often actually welcome a well-constructed audit even if it has been politically inspired!

For example, a therapeutic community, under threat of closure, recently audited the cost per year of their clients and then found out the cost of each of them to the community in the year prior to admission—hospitalisations, prison sentences, probation, etc. They were able to show that their charges, although expensive, were actually considerably less than the cost to the community, and they were given a three year reprieve.

◆ EXERCISE 3.2: Adding Practical Concerns to Your Topic Areas

Reconsider your topics in Exercise 3.1 and highlight those which meet any of the practical concerns described above. For example, label those which concern high cost areas with HC, local concern LC, those of interest to your team INT, and so on. When you finish doing that, chances are several topic areas will stand out as having one or more points highlighted. Hopefully, some will be under *Structure*, some under *Process* and some concerned with *Outcome*. From this you can prioritise the topics, perhaps beginning with *Structure* and moving on towards *Outcome*.

Finally, choose three topic areas around which to design your first audits.

CHAPTER FOUR

The Methods of Audit

THE AUDIT CYCLE

Figure 4.1 shows the simplest and most common version of the cycle which describes audit methodology. It presumes that you will always be setting standards for care, collecting data about how well you are meeting those standards, monitoring this data, and deciding what you will change about your practice as a result of what your data show. You then audit your practice again, to see that the changes you have introduced have made the difference you hoped for. In fact, with this model it looks as if you would go on auditing the same thing for ever.

However, life is never simple. For example, this type of cycle doesn't fit all audit methods nor show enough of what is involved. For a start, it makes no mention of selecting a topic (Chapter 3), and most people involved in audit agree that this is the part where it is crucial to get right. In this sense it needs emphasising as much as any of the other steps.

Moreover, some audits bring about considerable useful change without first setting standards: You decide upon a topic and the data you will collect, and you use that data to get an idea of what is actually going on in your practice. For most of us, accurate information such as this is extremely rare, often surprising, and invariably leads to change. After collecting the data you may then decide to set standards for any changes in order to encapsulate the elements of your practice you decide are good.

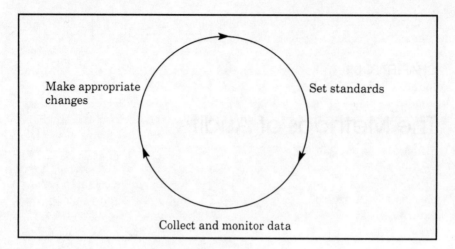

FIG. 4.1. The simple version of the audit cycle.

An example of such an audit was a survey of the satisfaction and preferred clinic times of psychotherapy clients, which led to the introduction of evening clinics. It was followed by a second satisfaction survey to check that satisfaction had increased. Another similar audit was of ECT in Britain (Pippard & Ellam, 1981). This found a variety of problems with the equipment, the methods, and the training of staff. This led to a Royal College of Psychiatry committee and DoH working group to recommend standards and ensure improvements.

How Many Times Around the Cycle?

In terms of how many times you might complete the audit cycle, two consecutive loops are generally seen as being enough. You will, however, want to re-audit a topic in a year or two to check that things are still going well, especially if there has been a frequent change of staff or conditions have altered significantly. Junior staff can usefully be given these re-audits as a project while they are with you, so the burden need not continually fall on you.

Pippard (1992), in describing the ECT audit mentioned above, said how, as a Mental Health Act Commissioner, he could see that frequently the earlier recommendations were not being followed. He says that it was clear that (p.621):

... it was exceptional for the doctor in charge of the ECT or the clinical tutor
to have provided adequate teaching for the junior doctors about ECT. The

drive to maintain standards stimulated by the 1981 report had not been maintained and the lack of audit of procedures was obvious.

Because of this, Pippard conducted a second audit 10 years later and found considerable improvement in the physical environment and in anaesthetic and nursing practice, but still less than effective equipment, little involvement from consultants, and unsatisfactory training and supervision of those who gave the treatment. He also found very large differences in use between districts.

Audit findings such as these are rich in terms of the possibility of producing change, and Pippard makes a number of recommendations, especially in terms of improvements in training and supervision, and of external audit.

THE COMMON METHODS OF AUDIT

The most common methods being used today include:

* **Casenote analysis (with or without standard setting).**
* **Reciprocal visiting or peer review.**
* **Criteria-based audits.**
* **Adverse occurrence screening/sentinel events.**
* **Patient surveys.**

The terms used in audit are still new enough to be somewhat flexible, and there's often overlaps between the methods, so don't worry if I call something by one name and you call it another. So long as the methods provide good data, that is all that matters.

Casenote Analysis

The most common way of looking at care over many years has been the discussion, via casenotes, of patients who suffer from similar disorders or who have had similar bad outcomes, such as a particular complication or death, for example, by suicide. The audit may be of a single patient, as often happened in psychiatry, or of an agreed number of patients chosen randomly within the group to be audited; for example, elderly falls on the ward in the last 2 months, the outcomes of 10 obsessional-compulsive patients being treated in the community, or a random selection of patients with manic-depression. Although casenotes are often reviewed in other audit methods (e.g. criteria-based or adverse occurrence screening), here **standards of care are not set prior to the collection of data; that is, you are not saying what should have been done until the casenotes are discussed.**

Exercise 4.1: Casenote Analysis

> As a group or as an individual, think about the benefits and
> disadvantages of this casenote method and note them below.

Benefits   Disadvantages

Comment: Some of the benefits and disadvantages that workshop groups
have brought up in the past are presented below. You may well have
different ones.

TABLE 4.1
Benefits and Reservations of Casenote Analysis

Benefits	Disadvantages
Prompts discussion about individual patients.	No objective standards have been set to judge the quality of care.
Shows up the problems in the quality of the casenotes.	Very time consuming.
Useful to follow a single case right through.	Difficult to randomise as casenotes often can't be found.
The detail can be educational for trainees and juniors.	If selection is random it may miss the important cases
	Junior staff complain it is sometimes used to criticise their care.
	It can become boring.
	It often focuses on negative outcomes.

Teams who are starting to audit will often use the casenote analysis
method to get the discipline of regular meetings and so forth set in place.

After six months or so, most people report finding the method limited and boring, though their casenotes have often improved enormously. In fact, some initiate a standard-setting for the quality of notes and audit the casenotes themselves (see p. 34 for such an audit).

Reciprocal Visiting or Peer Review

To some extent, all audit is peer review. However, as a method, this describes those audits where one group of professionals (an alcohol and drug service, a day hospital, a community home, or a group of psychologists or OTs, or psychotherapists) visits a similar group in another district or hospital or region.

Apart from the obvious usefulness of seeing how others tackle similar tasks, it barely counts as audit unless definite standards are set so that the data collected are in some way systematic. In practice, it is usually limited to audits of structure (see Chapter 3, p.19)—the quality of ECT units, of confidentiality and security, of waiting rooms, of OT facilities, and so on. As hospital and community services turn themselves into trusts, it seems inevitable that this method of audit will be limited to inter-regional visits where there is much less chance of competition!

Prospective and Retrospective Audits

Before discussing the other main methods, it is worth considering the issues surrounding whether to do your data-collection prospectively or retrospectively. In other words, what are the advantages of gathering your data by looking back over your practice for a certain period or for the last 50 patients, for example; or by beginning to collect the data from this point on; or by doing both concurrently.[1] Audits done by case note analysis will, as we have seen, always be retrospective, but there may be reasons why this is the best thing to do.

Footnote (1): Many texts refer to prospective audits—those which are planned from today to run into the future—as concurrent, because the data are collected concurrently with practice. I tend to use the term prospective because it is used in the same sense in research, and because it is possible to run retrospective and prospective audits concurrently—that is, at the same time. Using the terms in this way seems to lead to less confusion.

Exercise 4.2: Prospective and Retrospective methods of Audit.

Write down the advantages and disadvantages of the two methods		
	Prospective	**Retrospective**
Advantages		
Disadvantages		

Comment: The main advantage of prospective audit methods is that you know in advance just what data you will need to collect. This means you'll not have to search through piles of often badly written or badly kept files to discover that the particular bit of information was never recorded in the first place. You can design your data collection to be encompassed within one or two sheets of paper, which can even be coded for the computer as you go. Often the data sheet will be the first page of the casenotes, but you might want to keep it separately to avoid the risk of losing the notes.

The disadvantages of prospective or concurrent data-gathering become the advantages of retrospective methods. If you do a purely prospective audit there will be no baseline and so you'll not know what you have been doing previously and how much you change as a result of the audit. In fact, even if you don't set standards but merely begin to audit some aspect of care, there is no doubt that, in a prospective audit, you will change your practice simply by collecting the data. The moment we are being evaluated we improve our actions.

If you are used to doing research, then you'll find this difficult to accept, and you would be right—if this was research. But the whole purpose of audit is to improve our quality of care, so the fact that we have no baseline but we are still changing for the better just as a result of collecting data is fine! (This is discussed more fully at the beginning of Chapter 7).

Just the same, most people do like to know they are improving, and this might be a very educational aspect of audit. If it is, then you could at the same time **carry out a retrospective and prospective audit**, which should capture this change for you. For example, you could audit some aspect of the last 50 parasuicides using the same data sheet you use to collect, at the same time, the data on the next 100.

In fact, most audit cycles involve looking back to gather data on what has been happening (e.g. reasons for referral for psychological testing on a neurology ward); followed by the setting of criteria for what should happen (e.g. referrals will always take place if X, Y, and Z are present); followed by a re-auditing prospectively to see what happens now we have set the standards.

Although it is quite possible to audit retrospectively and prospectively at the same time using the same data sheet, in practice, you will find that prospective data sheets are more elaborate. The example on the following page is a retrospective audit which used the last 100 casenotes to look at whether they met the criteria set. Compare this to the data sheet in Table 6.1, a prospective audit from a psychiatric day hospital, looking at outcome and appropriateness of treatment. The latter will be described in much more detail in Chapter 6. It's referred to here to show the difference in the types of information collected by the two methods.

Criteria-based Audits

When you conduct a criteria-based audit, you define specific criteria and standards for meeting them which you then compare with your actual practice, either past or present.

You will often hear the terms "criterion" and "standard" used in various ways, often interchangeably. Here they are used as follows:

Criterion: The statement of care that is decided on in advance and that uses words and phrases which make it measurable; for example: "All new patients will be assessed by a psychiatrist and a nurse".

Standard The World Health Organization's definition of a standard is "The expression of the range of acceptable variation from a normal criterion". So the standard for the above criterion would be 100 per cent, since the word "all" has been included and no exceptions have been stated. If there were to be exceptions (e.g. certain types of patients need not be assessed), these would need to be spelt out in the standard.

Criterion Audit of Casenotes

Casenote No.

Date Range

	YES	NO	NA
1. Folder condition satisfactory:			
2. Diagnoses clearly recorded by medical staff on HMR1 or Diagnosis Proforma:			
3. Dates + Time clearly marked:			
4. All notes legible:			
5. Every entry in notes signed legibly by Doctor:			
6. All serious allergies/drug reactions recorded or 'Nil Known':			
7. History of PC, systems review, social history are all well documented:			
8. Medication on admission recorded (inc. dose):			
9. (a) Examination includes pulse and BP:			
(b) Examination includes weight and urine analysis:			
10. Investigations ordered are marked in notes:			
11. Consultants referrals documented appropriately			
12. Investigations appropriately filed in notes:			
13. Information told patients/relatives recorded:			
14. Discharge arrangements clearly stated in notes:			
15. Formal discharge summary typed within			
(1) 2 weeks of discharge:			
(2) 1 month of discharge:			
(3) 2 months of discharge:			
(4) 3 months of discharge:			
(5) letter present in folder:			
16. T.T.Os clearly stated with dosages:			

(Reproduced with permission Stockport Health Authority.)

Criteria-based audits use a method which to some extent nursing audit has been doing for some time: defining criteria and standards of the process of care and then checking that they are done. However, it can be directed much more widely than this and can certainly include audits of structures and, although more difficult, also those of outcome.

Although criteria-based audit is usually described as a method in itself, it is actually applied to most other audit methods as well. For example:

* it can be prospective, or retrospective via casenote analysis;
* it can look at the aspects of care leading to or reflecting good practice (which is what is usually meant by the method); or
* it can concern itself with adverse events.

Done well, it is the most useful method of audit since it involves a thorough discussion of what makes up good care, and the data can be collected and analysed in a way that is as systematic and critical as anything the Working Paper could have thought of.

In brief, what you should do for a criteria-based audit is to:

---

1. Select a narrow topic relating to patient care.
2. Discuss what would be the highest quality or best possible outcome of that care.
3. Use this discussion, or other sources, such as research, protocols of care, or other professional guidelines, and set criteria describing how you will know this care has been achieved.
4. Choose a sample (e.g. the last 50 patients, the next 50 patients, or both) and check the notes retrospectively, or the data sheet prospectively, to see if the criteria have been met in sufficient numbers to meet the standard.
5. Ensure that the discussion that follows data analysis focuses on the patients or situations where the criteria have not been met. This is not a witch-hunting session; most of the cases will have a particular explanation which might be a one-off, but might be significant enough to suggest changes in practice.
6. Re-audit as and when necessary; for example, when changes in practice have been made.

The Advantages of Criteria-based Audits

There are a number of advantages to this method. For example:
* It promotes clinical discussion.
* Decisions are reached about what is quality *before* the audit begins.
* Operational definitions ensure less ambiguity.
* Less threatening to trainees and junior staff.
* Less time-consuming in the long run.
* Audit can be repeated.
* The setting of criteria locally may relieve purchasers of the need to impose criteria and standards and audit them themselves.
* Locally set criteria may be able to be used in defence of legal actions (see Chapter 2, p.17).

Looking at these in more detail, the most important advantage is that the method **promotes an excellent discussion**; for example, centring around what is a good standard of care, an appropriate procedure, or a good outcome. This is not as clearcut as we might think. Different professional groups will have very different views about what they see both as a good way of approaching the care of a patient and what is ultimately a good outcome. For example, a doctor in an alcohol dependency unit might view compliance with Antabuse medication as a good outcome; whereas a clinical psychologist might see this as an inadequate outcome and outline adherence to a controlled drinking regime or to abstinence as being necessary.

If you feel that the care of patients in the mental health field is particularly difficult to identify since so many methods are appropriate, it is worth realising that other specialties and areas are much vaguer about such things than one might think. For example, I once ran a workshop for consultant obstetricians and in one of the exercises I asked them to draw up criteria for the appropriate use of forceps. They chose this topic because they thought they would be able to agree more easily on this than on others we had considered. In fact, there were eight members of the group and we ended up with eight different criteria for when each of them would use forceps. In such a situation, the discussion itself can bring about a change for the better, but this is augmented by the fact that the obstetricians then found it necessary to go back to the research literature to help them make a decision about forceps use.

This illustrates just how diverse clinical practice is, which might be fine because it reflects genuine uncertainty and a need for research. On the other hand, it might mean that some of the rather more outlying methods need questioning, particularly if an effectiveness audit shows they seem to produce less useful outcomes, or if they are more expensive but produce the same outcomes. It also shows how difficult junior staff might find it as they move between consultants and supervisors. Living with uncertainty is something we get used to in the mental health field, but it doesn't mean our practice cannot be audited.

Finally, it illustrates the fact that there may be as many opinions about the best approach to care within a professional group as there are between professional groups. This is particularly important in mental health audits because it may be all too easy to blame any lack of agreement on the multidisciplinary nature of the group, without appreciating that a similar situation can occur within any group of clinicians, even those from the same profession.

Nevertheless, if, because of the small number of staff involved, you are setting out to audit across health authority boundaries—for example, in a regional audit of child psychotherapy—then trying to agree criteria and standards in such a wide arena with limited time available might not be the best way forward. In this situation, adverse event occurrence (p.40) would be much easier, although again it may be politically more tricky because of the implications of making negative information public.

Another advantage of the criteria-based method is that the **quality of care is agreed before you start auditing**. This is in contrast to the early versions of casenote analysis where a group of professionals would simply discuss one or more cases and then say what they think should have happened. Stating what the quality should be means the whole process and especially **the data themselves are much less ambiguous**, and **less threatening to junior staff**. Moreover, it is less time-consuming in the long run because not only are the data faster and easier to collect, but also the meeting to discuss the results only needs to concern itself with those cases which did not meet the criteria.

Finally, because each criterion is written in such a way that it is clear to anyone what is meant by it—even those not part of the original discussion—**the audit can be repeated** and the results obtained can be meaningfully compared with those that came before. So a junior doctor or trainee on a short placement could be given the task of re-auditing within the time period they are around. Although it is good for them to be a part of the discussion that sets criteria in the audits they're involved in, it is not always possible, and this is a good compromise to given them the experience of travelling round the loop.

There is, however, still a price to pay for doing audit in this thorough way. The main disadvantage is the time that has to be spent agreeing the criteria and specifying them in such a way that everyone knows what it means and can judge whether it has been done or not. Since defining criteria and setting standards is such a key part of audit methodology, we shall spend some time considering how to do this.

Defining Criteria

To show the detail that this requires, consider the example at the beginning of this section: "All new patients will be assessed by a psychiatrist and a nurse". Even the word "new" would need to be defined, otherwise the person doing the audit would quickly be asking whether patients who've been well for the last three, five or ten years were new patients or not. Although it would depend on the purpose of your audit, you would most want to define how soon the patient was to be seen (e.g. within 24 hours of admission) and perhaps also by what grade of psychiatrist and nurse. You might end up with something like:

All those who are first-time patients or those whose last attendance was more than six months previous should be assessed by a psychiatrist of registrar level, or above, within 24 hours of admission.

And:

All those who are first-time patients or those whose last attendance was within the last two years should be assessed by a staff nurse within two hours of admission.

These criteria would usually be followed by a list of assessments so that the doctor or nurse could fill them in as they were done. If the criteria sound rather too strict, you may want to develop exceptions (see next page).

Exercise 4.3: Setting criteria

Look at the criteria set in the audit of casenotes on p. 34. Pick out the words that need further definition, and try defining them in such a way that an outsider could do the audit just as well as those who set the criteria.

It's not easy to define criteria in words so clear that everyone knows exactly what is meant the first time. In practice, it is often when you search for actual data that ambiguities and discrepancies are revealed. Because of this and because of the time it can take to agree on a criterion in the first place, it is as well not to set too many. How many you use will depend on the type of audit and whether you are going to have to search back through casenotes to see if criteria have been met. Depending on this, between six and twelve is the ideal range, although you can produce very useful data from even one criterion.

Setting Standards

A standard is the degree of compliance needed to meet a criterion. When this is 100 per cent (which is frequently the case), then your audit meeting after data collection will simply need to discuss those cases which have not met the criterion. If there are a number of occasions which are not meeting the criterion (in the above example, those who are not being assessed within 24 hours), you may want to add a list of exceptions, which become inevitable through the results you find. So you might have:

Criterion: *All those who are first-time patients or those whose last attendance was within the last six months should be assessed by a psychiatrist of registrar level, or above, within 24 hours of admission.*

Standard: 100 per cent.

Exceptions: Unless discharged within 24 hours.
Unless SHO assesses and discusses with Registrar.

In some audits, especially those of appropriateness and outcome, the standards will not always be implied from the criterion itself; for example, the standard for a successful outcome in brief psychotherapy for depression. In addition, your professional society or college may have laid down criteria or standards and you would rather use these. Although eventually you will use criteria and standards applicable to your local situation, **you could use any of the following to provide a place to begin:**

* **By a literature review of research (e.g. on outcomes) to see what standards are possible.** For example, standards might be indicated that a certain proportion of high expressed emotion (EE) families should lower their EE characteristics with education; or that this should lead to proportionally fewer relapses in certain groups of people diagnosed as schizophrenic. Similarly, the finding (Markman & Beeney, 1990; Newnes, 1993) that sending information about the clinic and its assessment

significantly increases attendance at the first appointment could be used to set the criterion that all new patients should have such information. A subsequent audit would simply check that this had been sent.

* **By college or professional society guidelines;** for example, on confidentiality of notes, or on the grade of staff required for the administration of ECT.

* **By a literature review of other audits which have published their standards and results** (e.g. from the journal *Quality in Health Care*).

* **By previously agreed local protocols of care.**

* **Patients' Charter** or other externally imposed criteria and standards.

It is difficult to set standards without access to up-to-date knowledge. Most hospitals or trusts have the ability to make computer-based searches of literature. If you don't have this facility it would be worth pressuring your audit committee to fund one. It would also be very worthwhile to subscribe to *Quality in Health Care*.

In practice there will be a number of areas where neither research literature nor national guidelines exist and you will have to set standards by discussion about current practice or by setting them at 100 per cent and then seeing what happens.

Adverse Event Screening/Sentinel Events

Part of the difficulty—but also part of the benefit—of criteria-based audits is that you have to define what is the optimum quality of care or the best possible outcome. Adverse event or adverse screening, on the other hand, looks at what is poor care or a bad outcome—what should take place but doesn't and what shouldn't happen but does. Sentinel or critical events are severe examples of adverse events.

An adverse event might be:

A clinic non-attendance rate of X per cent.
A suicide attempt by an outpatient.
An alcoholic patient in a detox unit becoming inebriated.
An anorexic inpatient taking laxatives.
A patient on lithium showing unacceptable levels of serum lithium in their blood.

An attack on a staff member.
Bedsores.
Readmission

A sentinel event might be:

A successful or serious suicide attempt while in hospital.
Brain damage or death after ECT.
Death from any cause while hospitalised.
A case of Salmonella poisoning.

The **advantages** of this method are that it is easier to define and to count negative aspects of care than it is to define what is good care, since the former are usually unambiguous. The method also is perfectly suited for use right across a hospital or community unit setting. Its main **disadvantages** are that it doesn't provide the richness of discussion that occurs when you look at what is good care or a good outcome, and its negative focus will inevitably make it threatening to some people.

♦**Exercise 4.4: Identifying Adverse or Sentinel Events**

List those events that would be adverse or sentinel to patient care *in terms of your professional group.*

Patient Surveys

Patient surveys, which have long been a part of research and of quality initiatives, ask the patients various questions about their perceptions or opinions on various aspects of their care. For example:

> Patient satisfaction.
> Needs assessment.
> Acceptability of services provided.
> Quality of life.
> Usefulness of particular communications.

Patient surveys are conducted by either questionnaires or interviews.

An interview survey:

* will ensure a much higher proportion of respondents, and
* will provide rich and detailed data.

However:

* it is very costly because of the time spent interviewing and then coding the responses.
* building up a valid and reliable coding system requires extra expertise if it is to be meaningful.
* patients may feel less likely to complain in an interview situation.

A questionnaire survey:

* is relatively cheap,
* can use previously constructed valid and reliable measures, and
* is anonymous.

However:

* response rates are notoriously low, even when self-addressed envelopes are provided.

Patient Satisfaction

The main problem with patient satisfaction surveys is that it is very difficult to get patients to declare themselves dissatisfied. However, Baker and Whitfield (1992) compared a group of patients who had recently changed GPs (without changing addresses) with a group who had not changed doctors. This showed that, although the levels of satisfaction in the former group still looked quite high, they were significantly lower than those in the latter group. It seems clear from this that we are looking for relative satisfaction, rather than satisfaction versus dissatisfaction, so the small dips you see in the mean scores of various items are more important than looking for any major cause for concern.

Choose your survey instrument by looking through some of the research literature available on this topic, rather than by inventing your own questionnaire, though you may well want to add a few points to reflect local situations. For example:

	Extremely dissatisfied					Extremely satisfied
How satisfied are you with:						
Creche facilities	1 2 3 4 5 6 7					
The timing of clinics	1 2 3 4 5 6 7					

A literature review will show you which are the most valid and reliable measures for your particular situation, and may also provide standards should you need them; for example, what level of satisfaction should you expect from what type of patient, given previous research findings. However, in reality, most people conduct surveys without first setting standards; what is revealed by the data you get leads you to set new or improved criteria and standards of care.

Choosing Your Method

There is no one right method for audit. Your choice will depend very much on local circumstances: availability of help, computing, access to patient administration systems (PAS) or other central data, whether you are working in a team or in a fairly isolated way. The following summary of points made in this chapter should help you decide on a method.

* Casenote analysis, done as systematically as possible, is a useful first method in order to get the process of audit underway, and to improve the quality of casenotes.
* Retrospective audits will be necessary if you are using casenote analysis, whether with or without setting criteria.
* Adverse event audits can be continuing while you are doing other types, since they can be performed prospectively and their topics are easily defined but also crucial to patient care.
* Criteria-based audits, done with tact, are a good way for teams to air different opinions about care and come to some useful agreement.
* Prospective criteria-based audits and adverse occurrence screening are better methods for audits conducted by trainees, since there should be much less ambiguity involved.

* As soon as your audit machinery and process is functioning, tackle a criteria-based audit, first aiming at structure, then process, then outcome.

♦Exercise 4.5: Choosing Your Audit Method

Taking the three priority topics you decided upon at the end of the last chapter, choose a suitable audit method for each. Decide also: whether it is to be prospective or retrospective; the population and time limits of your audit; and who will collect the data.

The following page sets out an action plan for audit. This will help you to design your audit, making sure you've asked all the necessary questions before you begin.

Audit Action Plan

1. Topic Area

2. Quality Area

3. The question I want to address

4. The purpose of asking the question/conducting the audit?

5. Who needs to be involved?

6. The Method:

   Prospective or Retrospective

   Population

   Setting criteria and standards first? YES/NO
If YES, how will criteria and standards be set?

Give examples

   What will the data be?

   How long will data be collected? _____

   Who will collect the data? _____

   How will the data be analysed?_____

   _____

   How will I feed the results back into my practice?

CHAPTER FIVE

Sources of Data

TYPES OF DATA

Once you have chosen a topic and a method for your audit project, the information that you will use for data will usually be obvious. For example:

* If you are **simply gathering information to find out what is happening** (e.g. how many clients are presenting with problems associated with early sexual abuse, and how are they being dealt with), then your data will be frequencies, perhaps categorised into various groupings, such as different clinics or types of referral.

* If you are using a **criteria-based** method, then your data will be the proportion of times you meet/do not meet each criterion.

* If you are using **adverse event screening** without setting standards (e.g. if you are simply gathering data on the number of attempted suicides in outpatients), then your data are simple frequency statistics, as described above. If, however, you are setting standards for adverse events—which will almost always be 0 per cent as they should never happen—then the data that matter will be the shortfall and your next audit would be to investigate why this has happened.

* If you are conducting an outcome **audit or a survey**, then your data will come from a data sheet or questionnaire (see Table 6.1, p.63), perhaps a well-validated one, perhaps one you have created yourself, within your professional group or as a multi-disciplinary group. (This is discussed in detail in Chapter 6.) In chronic conditions, this outcome (e.g. medication compliance, pain, carers' health, client satisfaction) will be taken at various intervals; whereas in acute conditions, the outcome measures will usually be pre-treatment, just at the end of treatment and at some time in the future as a followup. The data might be in the form of a mean symptom score, a target problem score, or a frequency score; for example, the number of independent activities on discharge.

* A final source of data, which might be used alone or might complement any of the others, is the hospital or community statistics that are being kept regularly; for example, resource management systems will show the number of days in hospital, and some systems for patient coding (for example, Read diagnostic codes) can be used to provide quite detailed information about patients, including family and social functioning. Other areas for useful statistics would be patient administration systems (PAS), casemix, district statistics, complaints register, and so on. The points made in the section on background data (p. 50), are very relevant to these data.

In practice, you will probably use a number of types of data in one audit (such an audit is described in detail in Chapter 6, p. 62). We will now look more fully at these data sources.

CRITERIA-BASED AUDITS

The principal data of all criteria-based audits is simply the percentage of "NOs" recorded on your datasheet, whether collected retrospectively from the casenotes or from a prospective datasheet.

For example, if occupational therapists decide to audit the activities of daily living (ADL) as an outcome of a rehabilitation programme, their data will simply be the percentage of patients who were still dependent in the target ADL activities which have become the criteria of a good outcome. For example:

Criterion: Can dress him/herself YES/NO

Since it can be argued that one is either dependent or independent, the percentage that matters is that representing the NOs, and these patients would then be looked at more closely. If you had set a standard for yourselves (e.g. of 75 per cent), then you might only be interested in considering the data further if you failed to meet that standard.

Very useful information is gathered by this type of audit data, and the fact that your attention is only directed towards the (usually) smaller proportion of cases where the criterion has not been met saves considerable time. Nevertheless, audits are expensive to carry out, and you might want to glean a little more information from the activity than this very simple method of data collection and analysis allows. A useful addition would be to ask for a reason whenever the criterion has not been met. Thus:

Criterion: Can dress him/herself YES/NO   If no, give reason

This will give you much richer data to work on in the meeting to discuss results, and so enable you to bring about change more easily. It will also provide you with a list of exceptions to your criterion which will enable you to meet standards with more accuracy in future.

Other examples of this way of using data would be:

* Percentage of times that criteria for discharge letters are unmet.
* Percentage of times that appropriate procedures are not followed in ECT administration (Pippard, 1992).
* Percentage of patients kept waiting more than half-an-hour in a clinical psychology clinic.
* Number of hours exceeding the criterion for CPN travelling time.

If these audits produced a very small proportion of unmet criteria, then the "Reasons Why Not" could simply be discussed at the meeting. If the proportion was expected to be large, then it might be necessary to classify these reasons into categories in order to understand what is actually going wrong; for example, whether excessive waiting time was due to the clinician's timetabling, late arrival of the ambulance, late arrival of the patient, and so on.

In retrospective audits, the information which provides this data may be found (perhaps after laborious search) in the casenotes, and then entered on your datasheet. In prospective (concurrent) audits, it will be entered at the time.

Exercise 5.1: Sources of Data

> Using the above examples, say whether your data collection would be retrospective or prospective, and the source of information you would use to get it.

Audit	Retrospective/ Prospective?	Source of Information
ADL		
Discharge letters		
ECT procedures		
Waiting times		
CPN travelling time		

Comment: Here are some suggestions for gathering data on these criteria-based audits. You may well have thought of others.

Audit	Retrospective/ Prospective?	Source of Information
ADL	Prospective	Data sheet on assessment
Discharge letters	Retrospective	Casenote analysis of letter
ECT procedures	Retrospective	From casenotes to datasheet
	Prospective	Straight onto datasheet
Waiting times	Prospective	Appointments datasheet at front of notes: delay plus reason with box to tick if >30′
CPN travelling time	Retrospective & prospective	From Kohner data & travel claims or data sheet

SOURCES OF INFORMATION FOR BACKGROUND DATA

Because it is an essential feature of audit that it reflects your local practice, it is a good idea to collect background data on your patients so that the local picture reflects the differences which distinguish them from those using other services in the area. **This is crucial if purchasers are to judge and use audit information in a useful manner.** For example:

* You need to know something about the socio-economic health of your patients—if they live in poverty or with no social support, or under environmental threat, for example, you might expect a worse outcome than if they were affluent; and you might expect

a larger proportion of "Did Not Attends" (DNAs) if your surrounding population has a poor public transport system.

* You need to decide upon and incorporate in your notes some measure of the **severity of the presenting problem**:

(a) The length of time and number of recurrences of the condition will give you a measure of chronicity.

(b) A validated outcome measure (see the next section) can be used at the initial assessment, since this level of symptoms is an important description of your group of patients. It can, of course, also be used again at discharge to judge the effectiveness of therapy.

(c) A reliable and valid general measure of psychological health, such as the General Health Questionnaire (Goldberg, 1978) can be used so you can compare your population with others, both general community samples and psychiatric samples (see p.55 for more detail).

These data can then be used for all the audits you undertake.

OUTCOME MEASURES

Because of the need in the United States of psychiatry, psychology, and in particular psychotherapy, to prove to medical insurance companies that the work of those involved makes a significant difference to the mental health of clients and patients, the 1960s and 1970s saw a vast increase in the sophistication of research methods and the reliability and validity of instruments with which to measure change. For example, by the 1980s, because of the results of several meta-analyses, we could say with hand on heart that psychotherapeutic interventions work—that they are significantly better than no treatment. The last decade in psychotherapy research has been driven much more by understanding who benefits most from which types of therapy, rather than just looking at overall effectiveness; which therapists are best for which clients; what is most helpful within therapeutic contact with patients, and so on.

The principles and instruments developed for the evaluation of psychotherapy can be used for most of the audits designed to look at the effectiveness of mental health services as a whole; in fact, instruments such as the Symptom Check List (SCL), described next, were designed for psychiatric services originally.

The SCL-90 and SCL-18

This 90-item Symptom Check List was devised by Derogatis and colleagues in 1973. Although quite long, it encompasses a number of scales, such as anxiety, depression, obsession-compulsiveness, hostility, psychosis, paranoia, and so on. This makes it a useful screening and assessment instrument in its own right; in addition, it is particularly sensitive to showing change in symptom levels, which is just what you want in outcome audits or research. It has been used in the United States as the recommended instrument for nearly 30 years, and now is being used increasingly in mental health services in the United Kingdom, so there is a growing amount of outcome research and audit studies available for when you set your criteria and standards of outcome. There are two shorter versions of the SCL; the briefest (Barkham et al., 1993) having only 18 items.[1] Although you gain in terms of speed of completion with this shorter version, you no longer have the scales which form mini-outcome measures in themselves. However, it is being used with increasing frequency, has been validated in this country, and is not copyrighted, unlike the SCL-90.

Measures for Depression and Anxiety

The **Beck Depression Inventory** probably remains the most used world-wide. This is partly because, with so many reported studies having used it, it provides a useful comparative measure for your own patients. However, the **Hospital Anxiety and Depression Scale** (HAD: Zigmond & Snaith, 1983) is being used increasingly in the United Kingdom, and has the benefit of having much more acceptable wording for patients. Another measure of anxiety which has been widely used is Spielberger's **State-Trait Anxiety Inventory** (Spielberger, 1983).

General Health and Quality of Life

For some treatments, it might be useful to use a general measure of health, such as the health questions from the General Household Survey, or the **Nottingham Health Profile** (NHP: Hunt et al., 1981), which is a well-validated measure of health status. Its dimensions cover physical mobility, pain, emotional reactions, energy, sleep disturbance, and social isolation. The **Functional Limitations Profile** (FLP: Patrick & Peach, 1989) also has both physical and psychosocial dimensions—mobility, body

---

[1]This short version is obtainable as Memo 1419 from MRC/ESRC Social and Applied Psychology Unit, University of Sheffield, S10 2TN, 0742 756600.

care, ambulation, housework, pastimes, emotions, alertness, and social interactions. The SF-36 is similar and is being used increasingly, especially in primary care (Ware & Sherbourne, 1992). These measures are often preferable to earlier ones, such as the **Activities of Daily Living** (ADL: Katz et al., 1963) or the **Barthel index** (Mahoney & Barthel, 1965), since they are completed by the patient rather than requiring a trained observer. They both show change well, but differently depending on the dimension (Fitzpatrick et al., 1992), which could be a problem for audit.

Quality of life is a very complex area, and an enormous number of scales have been designed. The important point seems to be that generic scales are not so useful as those that cover your particular area. It is beyond the scope of this book to go into the scales, but an excellent reference is *Measuring health: A review of quality of life measurement scales* (Bowling, 1991).

Measures Specific to Other Conditions

There is an enormous number of other useful measures which can be used for specific problems areas, such as eating disorders, interpersonal problems, substance abuse, expressed emotion in the families of people with schizophrenia, elderly functioning, and so on. There are also those suitable for demonstrating change after specific interventions, such as marital or family therapy, occupational therapy, and group therapy. A literature search will reveal the best one for your specific area. In addition, the **Outcomes Project at the Nuffield Institute of Health at the University of Leeds** is a depository for literature on outcomes of all kinds of health care and all types of disorders, and provides an information service on what is available and its quality. In addition, the DoH has commissioned the same group to produce Effectiveness Bulletins on various topics. These are to be circulated to purchasers and providers and should help in the setting of standards.

Personal Questionnaires (PQs)

At the first assessment or perhaps during the first session with the key worker (if you use that system) or therapist, you can, with the help of the patient, create a questionnaire using statements by the patient of the problems they most want to change. This should be a maximum of 10 problems and a minimum of three, and should include some which are more easily resolved than others just in case the patient sees assessment at least partly as a reflection of whether they're able to do well rather than whether you're able to help them! Figure 5.1 is an example of a personal questionnaire statement set down in a patient's own words:

The trouble with my son	0	50	100
My headaches	0	50	100
My bouts of anger	0	50	100
My feelings of depression	0	50	100
My hatred of Mondays	0	50	100

FIG. 5.1. An example of a personal questionnaire.

The patient completes the form by marking the scale in the relevant place as often as you both decide. It is useful for clinical work to complete them at least weekly, but for audit, it will be enough if you get at least three completed during the baseline period (before the first actual therapy session), even if it is one a day. The mean, or average, of these three will be your intake measure, and you'll take another three in the month following treatment and then again at some predetermined followup. This should be as long as possible, balanced against the need not to lose track of too many people—six months and two years is excellent if you can manage it.

Outcome Measures for Multidisciplinary Teams

There is no better way of getting to know what other people in your team do in their job than by asking them what aspect of functioning they would expect to change in patients as a result of their treatment: not what they expect to *do*, but what they expect to *change*. By discussing these in the type of detail necessary to create an instrument for auditing overall change, you will probably learn more about each other's practice than you would over the years spent working together.

You could use this discussion to work towards creating a joint outcome measure, using the relevant professional instruments where appropriate. Alternatively, you could use a general one like the SCL-18 to show overall change, alongside more specific assessments, related to the problem or to your intervention, or simply the patient's personal questionnaire.

♦ **Exercise 2: What should change?**

> Think about your client group and what changes you hope your professional involvement will bring about in them. Some of these changes may be general to all clients, and some may be more specific. In a third column note down which instruments you will use to measure these changes.

General Change   *Specific Change*   *Measure*

THE GENERAL HEALTH QUESTIONNAIRE

This questionnaire was designed for use as a community screening instrument (Goldberg, 1978). **It is not a change measure** and so is not suitable for outcome audits, but it is useful as a descriptive tool for showing the general level of psychiatric distress in the patients seen in your service or your department. For example, you might use it to see whether the ethnic proportions appearing at your clinic are representative of the proportions within the local population.

The GHQ comes in four versions: 60, 30, 28, and a 12-item version to provide a mean overall measure of distress (using Likert scale scoring with items scored 0, 1, 2, 3), or of "psychiatric caseness", where scores in columns 1 and 2 are not counted, and scores in columns 3 and 4 are counted as one point each. Therefore, using the GHQ-12, you would have a maximum score of 12 using the second measure. The most valid cut-off for caseness is three or above, but some people recommend using four or above to avoid false positives. In chronic populations it has been suggested that you count the second column ("About the same as usual") as one rather than zero.

PATIENT SATISFACTION

Although there have been some doubts expressed as to whether patient satisfaction is an outcome measure or a process measure, most people consider that asking the user and the one who pays what they thought of the service is not unreasonable. Although many people argue that patients do not have sufficient knowledge or expertise to judge the technical side of effectiveness, there are some aspects of quality, such as acceptability of treatment, which only they can comment on.

In mental health services, it may seem less controversial than in other specialties to gather the patient's opinion on these technical aspects as well. In fact, that is what we are doing when we use self-completion questionnaires such as the SCL-90. Even in other specialties, there is some evidence that patient satisfaction can affect outcomes, either via issues like compliance and attendance at clinics, or directly in terms of a positive change in symptoms (Fitzpatrick & Hopkins, 1983).

Measuring Satisfaction:

Patients generally always seem to score high on satisfaction, even when we know that the outcome was not as good as it could have been. This affects validity, in that we don't really know that it is satisfaction that we are measuring, and it affects reliability in that the scores tend to bunch so closely together at the top of the scale, it's hard to distinguish the dissatisfied from the satisfied.

Nevertheless, by demonstrating differences in satisfaction between those who had changed their GP but not their address and those who hadn't changed, Baker and Whitfield (1992) have shown that you can demonstrate validity. Also Stiles et al. (1979) showed that, where communication had been objectively poor between a doctor and patient, subsequent satisfaction scores were significantly lower.

So it is possible to get it right. Remember:

* You are looking for relatively small differences or blips in your data to show dissatisfaction in different situations.

* Do use a standard instrument which has been shown to be valid and reliable. A literature search of the patient satisfaction area will show you what's available for your particular field.

One general measure for hospital care is that developed by the CASPE Research Project which is short (15 items) and computer-scored to allow for large numbers. Another is the 63-item **Patient Satisfaction Questionnaire** (PSQ) developed by Ware, Snyder, Wright, and Davies (1983) which has the following eight dimensions:

1. Interpersonal manner (interactions with staff).
2. Technical quality (competence of staff in the process).
3. Accessibility.
4. Finances.
5. Efficacy of maintaining or improving health..
6. Continuity of services.
7. Physical environment.
8. Availability of medical care resources.

Whichever measure you use, make sure it's multidimensional in this way, and that it uses a scale rather than simply a YES/NO answer. One scale that seems to work well has questions designed like this:

How helpful was your treatment? (for example)				
Very unhelpful	Quite unhelpful	Neither helpful nor unhelpful	Quite helpful	Very helpful
0	1	2	3	4

When Do You Measure Satisfaction?

It's true that, if you measure satisfaction at the end of treatment—when we might presume that things seem rather better—the patient is likely to report being satisfied even if every bungle possible occurred on the way. This is because they are glad the whole episode has ended. The instrument may therefore be more sensitive to dissatisfactions if you measure at intervals during care rather than just at the end. In chronic conditions, where there is no real discharge, then this is of course essential. Asking clients what could have been done to improve various aspects of their care (using items reflecting the above dimensions) may take longer to analyse, but will often produce much more useful data in terms of bringing about change.

CHAPTER SIX

Analysing Your Data

WHAT STATISTICS DO YOU NEED?

There needs to be very little, if any, complicated statistical analysis in audit. As we described in the previous chapter, most data will be in the form of frequencies and percentages. For this reason there is no need to have sophisticated statistical software, and many audits can be done with a good calculator.

Having said that, there are advantages to having a personal computer (PC) for the department or team, and this will become essential if you are dealing with large numbers of patients, and if you also want to use your data for research as well as audit. Having the potential to analyse data statistically in ways which might generate research papers is also often an incentive for some professionals to become involved where they might otherwise be reluctant.

Even without the intention to do research, there will be times when you want to be able to statistically analyse your data. For example:

1. You might want to know whether the frequencies you are seeing are what you would expect. To illustrate, if you know that the percentage of psychological disorders in Asian women shown locally in a community sample is 10 per cent representing 3 per cent of the total female population, and you are showing 1.2 per cent of your clinic population of women to be Asian, you might

want to do a chi-squared test to see if this difference in frequencies is statistically significant. Of course, you don't need to do this in audit—you can just look at it and decide that, whatever the statistical tests tell you, it matters to your team that you are not meeting this community need. You may decide that your standard for this is that you will be satisfied if you are reaching 75 per cent of the numbers suggested by the community survey. Details about the use of the chi-squared statistic and others referred to here will be found in any basic statistics book (e.g. Runyon & Haber, 1991).

2. Where you are using a scale rather than frequency data you might want to look at the differences between the means of two or more groups, and so apply an independent t-test or one-way analysis of variance. For example, you might wish to know whether the patient satisfaction scores are higher for those clients you are able to see in the one evening clinic you run compared to those who have to come during the day. You might also want to compare satisfaction scores by patient diagnosis to see whether certain groups are not seeing their treatment as useful as other groups.

3. You might wish to investigate whether there is a significant correlation between one variable and another; for example, do patients get longer treatment the older they are (or perhaps even the younger they are)? Are those with more severe symptoms seeing more experienced professionals? For this you would want the Pearson r statistic to see if the relationship was significant.

It is true that questions like these can sometimes be answered by eyeballing the data, but a statistical test will often give you more confidence in deciding, for example, that more serious patients are being seen by less experienced professionals, and that this should be changed.

Many good calculators provide these statistical tests, but a PC with a statistics package (such as SPSSX-PC)[1] will give you more than enough sophistication to enable audits to be presented quite well (although not as well as they will if you also have a graphics package), while at the same time allowing you to do research with the data should it prove adequate.

---

[1] Supplied by SPSS Inc, 444 N.Michigan Avenue, Chicago, Illinois 60611.

AUDIT COMPUTER PACKAGES

There seem to be rather more complaints voiced about computer packages specifically designed for audit, than favourable comments. Those who have gone without computers or who have invested in a cheap PC and some simple software have, on the whole, progressed considerably faster with audit than those stuck with software way beyond their needs and their computing capabilities.

However, there are some useful packages available which can quite easily be adapted for audit: D-Base3 or Smartware can be used as a total administration system for a department—sending appointment and discharge letters, keeping a diary, and also simple audit data. In fact, Smartware has linked up with Manchester Royal Infirmary's psychotherapy department to design PSYPAS,[2] a package which can be used for most audits, including assessments, and which will also generate appointment and discharge letters. It takes details on both patients and therapists, including the skills, specialties or areas of interest of the latter.

ANALYSING OUTCOMES

Although most audits are merely a matter of descriptive statistics, effectiveness audits—deciding whether patients have had an adequate outcome from your care—are often seen as much more complicated. Deciding whether a patient group has changed for the better is the cause of huge debate between researchers and theoreticians, especially if treatments are being compared.

Comparing treatments, however, will always be research and never audit. Audit cannot make these comparisons because it uses real patients and therapists who can choose (or at least influence) which type of treatment they receive or give, rather than being randomly allocated to one condition or the other, or matched for age and sex. They won't have nice, neat diagnoses either, as happens in research groups, and will show the whole range of severity and history. What audit can do is to see what was achieved in research, use that as the standard for local practice, and check how well we are meeting that standard (see Chapter 1, p.9)

---

[2]Details of the PSYPAS system to go with SMARTWARE administration system can be obtained from Gabriel Consultancy Ltd, 96 Wellington Road South, Stockport, Manchester SK1 3UH.

An Example of an Outcome Audit

To illustrate how you might set criteria and standards and analyse your data in an audit which looks at the effectiveness of your service, as well as other aspects of it, we'll consider in detail the audit of a psychiatric day hospital.

This building was in extremely pleasant grounds, close to the M1, staffed with an unusually highly trained and well-motivated multidisciplinary staff. It saw only "neurotic" patients, unlike the other day hospitals in the city which saw a much more mixed group. There was a "key worker" system, so everyone regarded themselves as doing some form of therapy.

Fears were circulating that such a pleasant spot must be a prime target for closure, and this was part of the encouragement (what I mean by political reasons for doing audit) for us to evaluate as a team how well we were doing. Like anyone involved in mental health who is not regularly auditing their work, we had no idea what this might produce, and undoubtedly most people were a little anxious that they might not be doing as well as they would like. One person refused to join in at all. There was some initial enthusiasm for an audit which compared our hospital with one of the other day hospitals, but we couldn't do that: even if we could have got them to join us in the audit, their patients were not remotely similar to ours, either in diagnosis, severity or poverty levels, and staffing and other resources were different too. So we needed a design which would just show how effective we were being.

Table 6.1 shows our data sheet for the audit. It was designed by the team as a whole and some aspects of it reflected particular interests. However, apart from the SCL-90 and BDI assessments listed in the last eight lines, the rest of the audit was largely descriptive, but extremely useful as we had quickly discovered that we knew almost nothing about our patients as a group.

The form was used as part of the initial assessment, so completing it took no longer than it had to fill in the previous admission sheet. It was completed in coded form: if the patient was female, a 1 would be written at the end of the line for SEX, and so on. This meant that the person putting the data into the computer (a simple IBM-compatible PC with SPSSX-PC on it) could do it at the rate of at least one per minute. The length of psychiatric history was used as a measure of severity; we coded the four main diagnostic groups that we saw, though this would have been better done more formally with an ICD9 diagnosis, for instance. (I have no idea, for example, where we put those with eating disorders!)

We were only interested in whether patients were on therapeutic drugs or not. This would let us know whether those without medication were patients with higher or different initial symptom scores to those with medication, and whether they were doing as well. This would lead on to an

TABLE 6.1

Audit Data Sheet: The Day Hospital

CLIENT NO.		_____
IN OR OUTPATIENT	(In = 1, Out = 2)	_____
SEX	(F = 1, M = 2)	_____
AGE		_____
LENGTH OF PSYCHIATRIC HISTORY IN YEARS	(0 = < 1 year)	_____
MARITAL STATUS	(Mar = 1, Single = 2, Div = 3, Wid = 5)	_____
LENGTH OF ATTENDANCE AT WDH	(in weeks)	_____
MAIN PROBLEM	(Depn = 1, Anx = 2, Obs = 3, Pers = 4)	_____
ABUSE	None = 1, Sexual = 2, Physical = 3)	_____
TYPE OF THERAPY	(Pt = 1, AMT = 2, Behav. Prog = 3, CBT = 4)	_____
DRUGS	(Not on any Drugs = 1, On Drugs = 2)	_____
THERAPY MODE	(Indiv. = 1, Group = 2, Marital = 3, Family = 4)	_____
THERAPIST NO.		_____
SCL AT ADMISSION		_____
SCL AT 3 MONTHS OR INTERIM SCORE	(Not at end)	_____
SCL AT END OF THERAPY		_____
SCL AT FOLLOWUP		_____
BDI AT ADMISSION		_____
BDI AT 3 MONTHS OR INTERIM SCORE	(Not at end)	_____
BDI AT END OF THERAPY		_____
BDI AT 3 MONTH FOLLOWUP		_____

audit where we would set criteria for the efficient use of medication. However, if we had been specifically interested in our frequency of using different types of drugs, we could have coded 0 for no drugs, and then, say, 1–6 for the major categories.

The principal type of therapy offered was coded (whether it was a behavioural programme, or psychotherapy, or so on). In addition, we could see whether a person was assigned to individual, group, marital or family therapy. This gave us data on efficiency in terms of therapist:client hours.

We wanted to know, in particular, whether people had suffered from sexual abuse when young. This was because we were beginning to notice the sudden rise in numbers of these people, perhaps due to media interest, but also because of the rarity with which this is recorded in the notes, and the difficulty of finding it when it is recorded. Actually getting this question asked in the first few sessions, we hoped, would help to stop these patients receiving inappropriate therapy.

Finally, during assessment we used the SCL-90 as a general measure of symptoms, and the BDI because the majority of our patients were depressed (see Chapter 5, p.52 for a description of these). We repeated them at the end of therapy and at six months' followup. We also gave the measures at about three months into treatment, to see how things were going.

In addition to these formal measures, the group began to use PQs with individual clients (see Chapter 5, p.53). Our psychotherapy groups were assessed using Horowitz's **Interpersonal Problems Scale** (Horowitz et al., 1988) and our OTs began to try out a range of measures to suit various forms of functioning. These weren't entered on the assessment sheets, although they could have been, and perhaps should have been once people felt more comfortable with the auditing process.

Most of our data were simply descriptive. We could now see the proportions of our patients who were depressed, the age groups we were seeing, whether staff members were seeing predominantly one sort of patient, the types of therapy we were giving, and whether the number of sexually abused women was rising. All this was extremely useful in planning our service, especially in terms of training and supervision.

The Analysis of Outcome Data

Having said that audit is not research, in terms of analysing our outcomes the day hospital staff actually used a research model for looking at effectiveness. Most people think of research models in terms of the classic controlled trial: you give one group a treatment and the other matched group no treatment, or a placebo, or some variation on that, and you compare the outcome to see if the treatment group has done significantly better than the others.

However, once research has shown you that a treatment is effective (e.g. as meta-analysis has in psychotherapy research), then you can use a model where you don't need to make such comparisons. In fact, many people argue that the drug models are not suitable for much of mental health research, especially if they presuppose we can match groups in ways that are probably simply not possible as they are in research into physical illness. The design we used was described by Jacobsen et al. (1984), and an illustration of its initial result is shown in Fig.6.1.

The horizontal axis is each patient's intake score, while the vertical axis is their end-of-therapy score or follow-up score (one or the other). If a patient comes in with a score of 120 and goes out with a score of 120, or comes in with a score of 45 and goes out with a score of 45, then they will be right on the diagonal, indicating no change. If they come in with a score

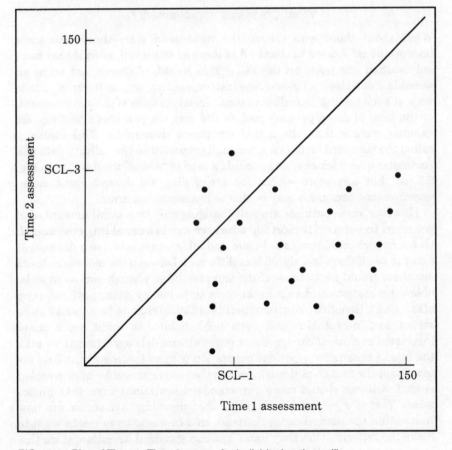

FIG. 6.1. Plot of Time 1–Time 2 scores for individual patients (I).

of 120 and go out with a score of 45 (or any other improvement) they will be on the lower right-hand side of the diagonal. If, as rarely but sometimes happens, they come in with a lower score than they leave with (in other words, if they deteriorate over the course of treatment), then they will be on the upper side of the diagonal.

The beauty of this system is instantly apparent: there are no averages of individuals, so you don't lose information; individuals are all represented by a dot, which you can identify as a person if you want to, but you can also colour according to diagnosis, or age-group, or whatever else you are interested in. Even at this stage, it is a clear and useful snapshot of your outcomes, and you can instantly see and investigate further those who have deteriorated.

What Counts as Improvement?

What about those who are on the right-hand side—those who show improvement? Are we to count all of them as improved, even if they have only shifted one point on the SCL? This would, of course, not be at all sensible. For a start, all measuring instruments are subject to error: results vary at each testing according to small idiosyncrasies of the environment, or the kind of day a person's had, or the way the pen keeps blotting, for example, rather than the actual symptoms themselves. This statistic, called the standard error (s.e.), is usually reported in the validity data of a particular questionnaire, and should be used to "widen" the lines, as in Fig. 6.2, so that any score within the broad diagonal doesn't count as an improvement because it may be due to measurement error.

However, some patients are still changing only by a small amount, and **we need to set a criterion for what we say is actual improvement**. Of course, we could just take before and after scores and use a dependent t-test to see if there is a significant difference between the means: chances are there would be, because if the sample's large enough you seem to be able to get statistical change in the short-term just by giving patients a cup of tea! But although we're interested in statistical change, because it's more robust and acceptable (and even publishable), in audit we're more interested in *clinical* change. Jacobsen et al.'s model suggests that we take the intake mean of our patient population (e.g. by looking at the first six months or the first 60 patients), and say that our criterion for improvement is that patients should move two standard deviations from that intake mean. This is a very strict criterion, often meaning that people are now well within the normal range. Instead, on a first audit you might want to make the criterion that they move just one standard deviation, since this is less threatening, but still puts them in a different population after treatment.

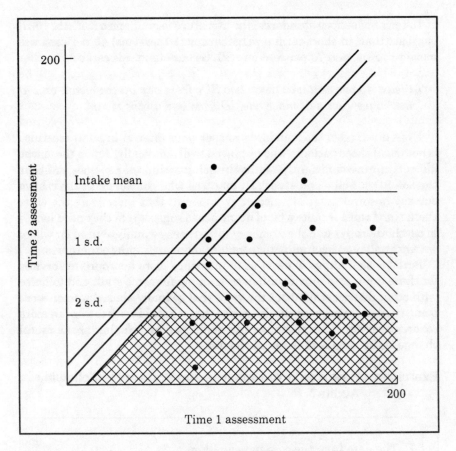

FIG. 6.2. Plot of Time 1–Time 2 scores for individual patients (II).

At the day hospital our effectiveness criterion therefore became:

By the end of psychotherapy our patients will have moved at least one standard deviation from our intake mean.

and we had to define "end" and set down our intake means and standard deviations on the SCL-90. Looking at Fig.6.2, the top horizontal line is the mean of our population; the next one down is one standard deviation (SD) below, and the lowest one is two SDs below. On the above criterion, anyone in the striped or cross-hatched area has improved because they have moved at least one SD. We can also judge how many have moved two SDs by counting the number in the cross-hatched area alone. These two groups are expressed as percentages of your total number of patients.

In terms of setting standards, the literature (e.g. Shapiro & Firth, 1987) suggests that, in short-term psychotherapy (16 sessions) 43 per cent will move two SDs, and 70 per cent one SD. So our standards can be:

At least 43 per cent will move two SDs from our intake mean, and at least 70 per cent will move one SD from our intake mean.

Even if you meet the standards you set, your interest in audit meetings is not on all those patients who improved so dramatically, but on those who did not improve sufficiently—either by being within the s.e. lines, or above the one SD cut-off—and especially on those who got worse. In the case of our day hospital, it was immediately apparent that these were the older clients (and there is quite a bit of literature to suggest that they need longer in psychotherapy), and the women who had been sexually abused for whom we were only just beginning to introduce more appropriate therapies.

Both these findings allowed us to introduce more appropriate services for these groups, to provide different training for some staff, and to liaise with other district staff about the ways that sexually abused women were being treated throughout the district so that we could work towards a more coherent service. This closing of the audit loop by bringing about useful change is the subject of the final chapter.

Exercise 1 : How Would You Analyse and Present the Following Audits?

1. The data from the case-note audit on p. 34.
2. A comparison of OPD waiting-times before and after the introduction of a new system.
3. An outcome audit of an outpatient clinic.
4. A criteria-based audit of bedsores.
5. An audit of travelling time for CPNs.
6. A quality of life audit for carers of people with schizophrenia, some of whom attend a local centre.
7. A communication audit of discharge letters to GPs of children attending a child psychiatric outpatients.

Comments:

1. This would simply be the percentage of casenotes which failed to meet any particular criterion. These percentages would be best expressed as a bar-chart for each criterion, so you could see at a glance where things were

not working too well. When you make changes as a result of your audit, you would then set out in bar-charts data illustrating the worst of the criteria last time next to how you have done this time. This should let you see the effectiveness of your changes.

2. This would depend on your audit design, but the simplest would be to keep a record of the number of people kept waiting more than 30 minutes (contrary to the Patients' Charter) at 30 minute slots during the day. You could show this as a line graph over the 8 hour period in order to see at what points there are build-ups. The followup audit, taken after the changes, could be mapped on to the same graph using a different line style, and this would show visually what improvements (or deteriorations) had occurred.

If you wanted a more detailed audit, then you would count the number of minutes past the appointment time each person is kept waiting, and plot the means of these for each time period. You could use a t-test to compare overall mean delay before and after organisational change, although the visual display of this data would probably be all that is required.

3. An outcome audit of an outpatient clinic (or of anything else) could be done by giving an appropriate psychometric assessment at Time 1 (or asking for a patient's target problems to be rated, or both), again at the end of treatment, and on followup, perhaps at one year. I would take the intake mean and standard deviation of the first two months, and set out my data in the way shown in Fig.6.2.

4. A criteria-based audit of bedsores would again be percentages expressed in the form described under (1). This could be used to see if national standards were being met.

5. An audit of travelling time for CPNs could simply involve a retrospective audit of Kohner data, but this would provide very little useful information. It would be more instructive to have a form which showed the destination and time taken for each trip, and each resulting visit, the reasons for it, and what the CPN considers to have been achieved. This is complicated and would need coding into categories to judge the types of reasons and the perceived usefulness of the visits, but it is the sort of situation where largely useless data has been collected for years and where audit could—if you were clear about the purpose of its collection—provide the basis for criteria for visits.

This would potentially be a good way for CPNs to be able to prioritise visits. However, by doing the audit prospectively in this way, there is little doubt that practice would change during the actual audit, so there would be less obvious change shown through re-auditing. Nevertheless, if you wanted to demonstrated change, you could use *t*-tests to compare the mean travel time (from Kohner data) or miles (from travel forms) after criteria were set up with that in the same period the year before.

6. A quality of life audit for carers of people with schizophrenia, some of whom attend a local centre, would initially be a descriptive audit showing the mean scores on the various sub-scales of the measure used. It could then go on to break these down so that the sub-group of carers' whose relatives attend the centre can be compared with the rest to see if this experience is particularly helpful (although you could not presume the two groups were equal). If research exists using the measure on a similar group to yours, you could use this to provide standards for your own carers (although you might not consider them high enough), and design changes to improve the areas where these standards are not being met.

7. A communication audit on discharge letters to GPs of children attending a child psychiatric outpatients, would best be addressed as a joint audit between the child psychiatry or psychology team and the GPs so that the latter could say what information would be most useful to them. In this way you would set up the criteria, and then simply audit 100 discharge letters (retrospectively and prospectively if you wanted to demonstrate change) to check that this had been done. The analysis and presentation would be as described in (1). (For a general discussion of how GPs and mental health services can work together see Wright (1991).) An example of a discharge letter for psychiatry follows.

DISCHARGE LETTER

_____HOSPITAL   DEPARTMENT OF PSYCHIATRY
    CONSULTANT _____

Dear Dr _____
I have pleasure in send you the following details of your patient who has just been discharged from this hospital.

Patient: Name ....
            Address:...
            Telephone: ....

Next of kin: Name: ....
                Address: ....
                Telephone: ....

G.P.   Name: ....
            Address: ....
            Telephone: ....

Hospital No.   .... Date of birth: ....
Admission date:...................................... Discharge date: ....

REFERRED BY:
1. self: 2. GP: 3. CPN: 4. Social worker: 5. Psychiatrist: 6. Police: 7. Other _____
ADMISSION: 1. Voluntary: 2. Section number _____

DIAGNOSIS _____
MANAGEMENT _____

PRESENT PROBLEMS: 1. Thought disorder: 2. Withdrawn: 3.Depression: 4. Anxiety:
5. Other comments: _____ 6. Work prognosis _____
DISCHARGE: by 1. Self: 2. Dr.
              to 1. Home: 2. Hostel: 3. Part III: 4. Sheltered: 5. Other _____

MEDICATION   Drug:_____Dose frequency: _____Qty: _____
              Drug:_____Dose frequency: _____Qty: _____
ADVICE:

Patient given shared care record: YES☐   NO☐

RISK FACTORS: 1. Lives alone: 2. Single parent: 3. Little family support: 4. Young children:
5. Divorced: 6. Recent bereavement: 7. Housing problems: 8. Social neglect: 9. No fixed
abode: 10. Multiple admissions: 11. History of self injury: 12. Drug/alcohol problems:
13. Poor compliance: 14. Other _____

OCCUPATION _____

FOLLOW-UP PLANS: 1. GP follow-up. Appt date _____
2. CPN _____ 3. Outpatient clinic appt. date _____
4. Occupational therapy _____ 5. Day centre _____
6. Retraining _____ 7. Rehabilitation _____
8. Social worker involved _____ 9. GP responsible for injections YES☐   NO☐
10. Other _____

SIGNED _____

Adapted from Essex et al. *British Journal of General Practice,* August, 1991

CHAPTER 7

Bringing About Change

THE EFFECTS OF GATHERING DATA

There is a phenomenon which psychologists have noticed and written about over the years: keeping a record of something that concerns or involves you—a diary of what you eat, a note of the times a child wets the bed, how many pain-killers you've taken—just the act of recording data seems to lead to improvements, whether by actually changing behaviour or by making your perception of it more accurate. The way it changes behaviour for the better is known as the Hawthorn effect: measuring workers' productivity in a factory was enough to improve it significantly, if temporarily, without introducing any of the planned organisational changes. Although it doesn't always last, its effects can be quite dramatic. For example, in an efficiency audit junior doctors were asked to record their reasons for out-of-hours X-rays; just by asking this, requests dropped from 698 to 493 during the audit period. So it's not surprising that aspects of care often change for the better during the audit, which is one of the reasons why audit stays distinct from research (see Chapter 1, p.9).

THE EFFECTS OF DISCUSSING CARE

Another reason why audit changes practice is that discussion between colleagues, sometimes for the first time, may reveal that our personal practice has some idiosyncrasies of which we were not aware previously.

For example, a group of psychiatrists knew their colleague was prescribing inappropriate antidepressants and had been doing so for years, but they did not feel able to tell him. It was only during a discussion of ways to improve prescribing, considering in detail the guidelines for appropriateness of different medication, that he realised his practice needed changing—and he changed.

Of course, he might not have changed. The role of the team in encouraging this is difficult, and most of what is written about audit tends to glide over what to do about consistently poor practice. Ultimately, it seems inevitable that the person's manager will need to be involved, probably via the unit's audit committee chairperson.

DECIDING WHAT NEEDS CHANGING

The audit activity as a whole is designed to demonstrate the areas which need to be changed. If you are conducting an audit without first setting standards, the necessity for change is sometimes not so obvious since what is good quality of care hasn't been decided upon in advance. Even here, however, you should be able to pick out aspects of your results which seem to be less appropriate or therapeutic than others, and you would then design criteria and standards around these points.

If you have set criteria and standards from the beginning, the areas which require change should be immediately obvious. Just by highlighting those items on your questionnaire where your practice, group or individual, has not met the standard you agreed upon will give you an ample agenda for discussion in your next audit meeting, and for bringing about further change.

Exercise 7.1: What Needs Changing?

You find that a criterion or standard you have set as a group has not been met—for example, compliance rates for medication in outpatients are lower than expected. Jot down some of the possible reasons for these discrepancies, and the general areas of change which might be necessary.

Comment: Your notes will probably have focused on at least five areas, such as:

1. Your practice may need changing. You might need to introduce further training, or a different routine to ensure compliance, or more frequent visits.
2. The patients' behaviour might need changing, which again inevitably means changing something in your practice; for example, by introducing written instructions, or by working more closely with the carers.
3. Management's assistance may be necessary to bring about structural changes; for example, by employing more CPNs.
4. There may be special reasons why this particular sample was different, in which case you will need to initiate another audit to check again.
5. The criterion might have been poorly worded. For example, it might have said that patient compliance should be "adequate" without defining precisely what this meant.
6. The standard might have been too high. For example, if you had a standard of 100 per cent for a criterion, as you often do, the audit might show that your particular local circumstances, or population, or staffing made that impossible, and that 80 per cent would be more realistic but still stretch you. Of course, you have to think very carefully about all the other possibilities before you decide on this particular change.

As you can see, one quite discrete audit can end up producing numerous changes, which in turn should be re-audited. If we look at the example of the day hospital audit (Table 6.1) and apply the above areas of change to that, most of our changes would be in the realm of providing extra services and arranging new training. In fact, we linked with an experienced woman from social services to begin groups with sexually abused women, as well as the with psychologists across the district who were dealing with this new influx, and began to meet together regularly for supervision, discussion, and support.

In today's health marketplace such joint enterprise might no longer be able to take place, certainly not without a transfer of funds. Worse, it is always possible that a difficult group like this who can often be patients of mental health services for years, may be seen by some services as too costly to treat in any in-depth way. This probably won't happen, but it is worth remembering that potentially it could, if, for example, you are telling a manager the overall beneficial results of your outcome audit. "And who's that group there?" he or she might rightly ask. "Why aren't they improving?"

In the day hospital audit we did actually lower our standards. Setting them to require a change of two standard deviations, as Shapiro and Firth (1987) had indicated, was fine as a goal to work towards. But many of our clients were considerably more disadvantaged in the rest of their lives than their research clients were, and so we decided on the additional standard, that 70 per cent should move at least one standard deviation, which seemed rather more realistic.

PRIORITISING CHANGE

When you have listed all the possible changes from your audit, prioritise them and write action plans for the top three. This might involve setting criteria (or new criteria), and these will need to be re-audited. Where criteria are clearly set, these re-audits can be done by a junior or a trainee as an audit project which will just fit their time with you and give them a chance to go once around the audit loop. If they can also be part of a criteria- and standard-setting exercise, so much the better.

In summary, practice changes:

* By the act of gathering the data itself.
* By discussing the question and the data with colleagues.
* By observing the results and deciding which areas require change and discussing how this might be achieved.

INVOLVING OTHERS IN CHANGE

While it is usually relatively easy to change aspects of one's own practice which are highlighted by audit results, improving clinical care usually involves a number of people: colleagues, juniors or trainees, other professionals, managers, and so on. Getting them to change their behaviour often needs new skills.

Exercise 7.2: Who Should Be Involved?

A group of psychiatrists audited the numbers of what they considered to be "inappropriate" referrals from GPs simply by counting all those they considered should have been better directed straight to clinical psychologists. They judged that 25 percent of referrals were inappropriate in this way. Spend a few minutes jotting down what you think they should do with these results.

Comment: However you answered this, the key expressions are **consultation**, or **participation** or **getting others on board**. There is no doubt that, if others are going to have to change as a result of audit, the more you consult with them, the more you encourage them to participate in the audit right from the beginning, and the more you involve them in the decision-making about necessary change, the better will be your chance of improving practice. Thus, you would have involved the GPs and the psychologists in setting the criteria.

(In a similar situation, orthopaedic surgeons saw their inappropriate referral rates drop by half after they had instructed GPs on when to refer direct to physiotherapy. They presumed these were now going as they had set out. Unfortunately, the GPs, who felt understandably irritated at being told what to do, were not referring patients to the physiotherapists as they had been instructed, but to the trust hospital down the road. Had the consultants spoken to the physiotherapists or audited with them, they would have picked up what was happening. Had they consulted the GPs and physiotherapists in the first place, the change they brought about would have been successful.)

Ideally, you will anticipate at the time you design your audit those who would be involved in future change, and so would encourage them to join you in designing it right from the beginning. We know from organisational psychology research that full participation in the decision-making process allowed to some workers is highly related to a lack of industrial problems and higher productivity. So, if you were designing an audit around waiting-times in outpatients' departments, you would ideally involve clinical, nursing, and clerical staff.

However, audit throws up surprises, and it will often result in the need for changes by others which you have not anticipated. For example, auditing the appointments system, as described above, might reveal a need to change the practice of ambulance drivers, and so they would have to be involved in deciding what should change and be part of the next audit. An audit of the efficiency of the procedure for discharge letters revealed that, in order to save the hospital some money, the post clerk was holding on to the letters until she had a "sufficient" bundle to make postage worthwhile—often for up to two weeks!

If you have to get others to change their behaviour to improve practice, then:

* Show them the results and ask them for their advice on how necessary change can best be achieved.
* When this has been agreed, both of you might want to set criteria and standards.
* Conduct a joint audit of adherence to these criteria.

GETTING MANAGEMENT TO CHANGE

As doctors, psychologists and other professional groups take on more and more management roles, as some of them become clinical directors or run trading agencies, for example, then the division between managers and health professionals will become less apparent. However, in the meantime, many staff tell me there is no point doing audit because managers will not pay for the changes shown to be necessary.

♦ **Exercise 7.3: Involving Managers in Audit**

> Think of ways to improve your chances in dealing with those who hold the purse-strings.

Comment: Involve them from the beginning by letting them know about the audit. They need to know about audits which might save money just as much as those which will cost money, especially when they are new to audit and its benefits.

* Give them regular feedback if it is a long audit.
* Make the results visually interesting, relevant and with not too much detail (though have this for back-up if necessary).
* Ask their opinion about what changes they would think were necessary.
* Try to have an idea of the costs which might be involved.
* If they do not have the money now, ask them what they would suggest you do as a compromise, or in the meantime. Try to fix a time to review the problem.

The same points apply in terms of dealings with the local audit committee, or with the Regional Health Authority: the more people feel involved and owning something of the audit, the more likely they are to want to become involved in the change process. Do make sure that you are well represented on your local audit committee, that you offer to discuss your audits with the local MAAG (the GPs' Medical Audit Advisory Group) to see if there is any chance of conducting joint audits, or at the very least to let GPs know how well you are doing; for example, with an audit news sheet.

Similarly, if you hold any sway with the local audit committee, then encourage them to include a manager as soon as possible. When this has been done, the committee invariably regards it as more of a help than a hindrance and you are much more likely to get necessary funding when the usefulness of audit is fully understood.

Every audit that you do will have an action plan with implications for someone to do something. It might be that one of the people that has to do something is a manager, in which case this will be recorded in the usual way. To some extent this becomes an audit of the management of audit, as you can check up on the times that managers have responded positively or negatively, and so on. Another essential record is whether the change will cost money or save money—and you could get your manager to help you work out how much. Again this is an audit of your audit activity, even though it's only tapping one dimension.

GETTING COLLEAGUES TO CHANGE

You will not get everyone to do audit and you will not always be successful in getting colleagues to change their practice as a result of audit findings. At the beginning at least, it is better to put your energies into working with those who want to change or those you really need to change, rather than with those who stick their heels in the mud or their heads in the sand, depending on your favourite metaphor.

Nevertheless, since audit in itself improves practice as well as providing educational opportunities, we need to encourage it wherever we can. This is likely to be increasingly important in the future where it is probable that, if we are not seen to be doing it accurately and efficiently, purchasers will find some way to conduct those audits themselves.

As mental health workers, you hardly need to be told that we do those acts for which we are rewarded and avoid those for which we are punished. If you are responsible for encouraging others to do audit, then it's worth working out just how you can reward people for taking part. One way often comes through the very act of doing audit itself—people frequently notice that they have finally been shown to be doing a good job. Seeing this demonstrated by data is much more reinforcing than just having a vague idea (or worse, vague doubts) about it, so make sure your group is as generous and as perceptive with pointing out and publicising the good aspects of practice which have emerged, as well as those which are not so good (Firth-Cozens & Storer, 1992). Holding meetings with other specialty groups or with GP referrers all encourages audit to be seen as an activity which is educational rather than persecutory and which does have real rewards in terms of improved care.

Remember when you are discussing audit that it is the changes you have made as a result, rather than the data itself, which is ultimately the most rewarding—so keep these changes carefully, and even publicly, recorded.

ACTIONS FOR CHANGE

You won't know that you are complying with change unless you are sure what changes are required. There are various ways to ensure that everyone is aware of this.

* At the end of each meeting's report, make an action plan (see Chapter 2, p.15). Write a list of required changes, who will be involved, and when they will be required to take some action.
* Make sure these changes are communicated to new juniors and trainees as they come into post, alongside a list of audits currently in progress, and of course relevant criteria and standards. This is sometimes done by getting them put into a looseleaf notebook, or by giving them a filofax sheet, or even a Psion organiser, depending on your level of sophistication.
* Make regular reports to your local audit committee of changes implemented. They will also play a role in following changes through.

EVALUATING CHANGE

If you have your changes clarified in the way described in the section above, evaluating their effectiveness will be much easier.

One way to do this is to travel the audit loop again, perhaps straight away, perhaps in six months or a year. This is particularly important if you have a high turnover of junior staff who will also need to have the audit and its findings explained to them, and to feel secure and involved enough to use the audit on themselves. You might even get newcomers to take over the next cycle of the audit, both to carry it on, to familiarise themselves with local criteria and standards, and to give them practice in carrying out audits.

IN CONCLUSION....

Audit can be frustrating and time-consuming, it's true. However, it can also be exciting and fun. As a team it will give you a better knowledge of your colleagues' ways of working than perhaps anything else you may do together. You travel more than the audit loop when you work together in this way but, done with your usual humour and tolerance, I'm sure you'll travel with enjoyment and real learning.

References and Bibliography

Baker, R. & Whitfield, M. (1992), Measuring patient satisfaction: A test of construct validity. *Quality in Health Care, 1,* 104-109.

Barkham, M., Hardy, G.E., & Startup, M. (1993). Development of a brief core outcome battery: Confirmatory analyses of short versions of the SCL-90R and the inventory of interpersonal problems. *SAPU Memo No. 1419.*

Bowling, A. (1991), *Measuring Health: A review of quality of life measurement scales.* Buckingham: Open University Press

Bull, A. & Firth-Cozens, J. (1991). *Medical audit in Yorkshire.* Yorkshire RHA Document.

CASPE (Clinical Accountability, Service, Planning and Evaluation Research Project) See Carr-Hill, R., Dixon, P., & Thompson, A. (1989). Too simple for words. *Health Service Journal, 99,* 728-729.

College of Speech & Language Therapists (1991). *Communicating quality: Personal standards for speech and language therapists.*

Department of Health (DoH). (1989). *Medical audit. Working Paper 6: Working for patients.* London: HMSO.

Derogatis, L.R., Lipman, R.S., & Covi, M.D. (1973). SCL-90: An outpatient rating scale: Preliminary report. *Psychopharmacology Bulletin, 9,* 13-20.

Donabedian, A. (1966). Evaluating the quality of medical care. *Millbank Memorial Federation of Quality, 44,* 166–208.

Essex, B.,Doig, R., Rosenthgal, J. & Doherty, J. (1991).The psychiatric discharge summary: A tool for management and audit. *British Journal of General Practice, 41,* 332–334.

Firth-Cozens, J. (1992). Building teams for effective audit. *Quality in Health Care, 1,* 252–255.

Firth-Cozens, J. & Storer,, D. (1992). Registrars' and senior registrars' perceptions of their audit activity. *Quality in Health Care, 1,* 161–164.

Firth-Cozens, J. & Venning, P. (1991). *Audit officers: What are they up to?* British Medical Journal,

Fitzpatrick, R. (1990). Measurement of patient satisfaction. In A. Hopkins & D. Costain (Eds.), *Measuring the outcomes of medical care* (pp.19-26). London: Royal College of Physicians.

Fitzpatrick, R. & Hopkins, A. (1983). Problems in the conceptual framework of patient satisfaction research: An empirical investigation. *Sociology of Health & Illness, 5,* 297-311.

Fitzpatrick R., Ziebland, S., Jenkinson, C., & Mowat, A., (1992). Importance of sensitivity to change as a criterion for selecting health status measures, *Quality in Health care, 1,* 89-93.

Goldberg, D.P. (1978). *Manual of the General Health Questionnaire.* Windsor: NFER.

Horowitz, L.M., Rosenberg, S.E., Baer, B.A., Ureno, G., & Villasenor, V.S. (1988). Inventory of interpersonal problems. Psychometric properties and clinical applications. *Journal of Consulting & Clinical Psychology, 56,* 885-892.

Hunt, S.M., McKenna, S.P., McEwen, J., Williams, J., & Papp, E. (1981), The Nottingham Health Profile: Subjective health status and medical consultations. *Social Science and Medicine, 15a,* 221-229.

Jacobson, N.S. & Truax, P. (1991). Clinical significance; A statistical approach to defining meaningful change in psychotherapy research. *Journal of Consulting & Clinical Psychology, 59,* 12-19.

Jacobson, N.S., Zollette, W.C., & Revenstorf, D. (1984). Psychotherapy outcome research: Methods for reporting variability and evaluating clinical significance. *Behaviour Therapy, 15,* 336, 352.

Katz, S., Ford, A., Moskowitz, R., Jackson, B., & Jaffe, M. (1963). Studies of illness in the aged: The index of ADL: A standardized measure of biological and psychological functioning. *JAMA, 185,* 914-919

Mahoney, F. & Barthel, D. (1965). Functional evaluation: The Barthel index. *Maryland State Medical Journal, 1,* 61-65

Markham, P. & Beeney, E. (1990). DNA rates and the effect of opting in to a clinical psychology service. *Clinical Psychology Forum, 29,* 9–10.

Maxwell, R. (1984). Quality assessment in health, *British Medical Journal, 288,* 1470–1472

Merrell, A., Patel, R., & Taylor, J. (1991). *Audit for the therapy professions.* Keele: Mercia Publications.

Newnes, C. (1993). A further note on waiting lists. *Clinical Psychology Forum, 53,* 33–35.

NHSME (1991). Framework for nursery services. London: Department of Health.

Oppenheim, A.N. (1968). *Questionnaire design and attitude measurement.* London: Heinemann, Educational Books.

Parry, G. (1992). Improving psychotherapy services: Applications of research, audit and evaluation, *British Journal Clinical Psychology, 31,* 3-19.

Parry, G. & Watts, G.N. (1989). *Behavioural & mental health research: A handbook of skills and methods.* Hove: Lawrence Erlbaum Associates Ltd.

Patrick, D. & Peach, H. (1989). *Disablement in the community.* Oxford: Oxford University Press.

Pippard, J. (1992). Audit of electroconvulsive treatment in two National Health Service regions, *British Journal of Psychiatry, 160,* 621-637.

Pippard, J. & Ellam, L. (1981), Electroconvulsive treatment in Great Britain, *British Journal of Psychiatry, 139,* 563-568.

Powell, G. (1989). Selecting and developing measures. In G. Parry & F.N. Watts (Eds.), *Behavioural and mental health research: A handbook of skills, Vol. 7, Methods.* Hove: Lawrence Erlbaum Associates Ltd.

Royal College of Psychiatrists (1989). The Royal College of Psychiatrists: Preliminary report on medical audit. *Psychiatric Bulletin, 13,* 577-580.

Runyon, R.P. & Haber, A. (1991). *Fundamentals of behavioural statistics.* Maidenhead: McGraw-Hill.

Shapiro, D.A. & Firth, J. (1987). Prescriptive v. exploratory psychotherapy: Outcomes of the Sheffield Psychotherapy Project. *British Journal of Psychiatry, 151,* 790-799.

Spielberger, C.D. (1983). Manual for the State-Trait Anxiety Inventory, STAI. Palo Alto, CA: Consulting Psychologists Press.

Stiles, W.B., Putman, S.M., Wolf, M.H., & James, S.A. (1979). Interaction exchange structure and patient satisfaction with medical interviews. *Medical Care, 17,* 667-679.

Ware, J.E. & Sherbourne, C.D. (1992). The MOS 36-item short-form health survey (SF-36): Conceptual framework and item selection. *Medical Care, 30,* 473–483.

Ware, J.E., Snyder, M.K., Wright, W., & Davies, A.R. (1983). Defining and measuruing patient satisfaction with medical care. *Evaluation and Program Planning, 6,* 247-263.

Wright, A.F. (1991). General practitioners and psychiatry: an opportunity for cooperation and research, *British Journal of General Practice, June,* 223-224.

Yates, B. (1980). *Improving effectiveness and reducing costs in mental health,* Springfield, IL: Thomas.

Yates, B. & Newman, F.L. (1980). Approaches to cost-effectiveness analysis and cost-benefit analysis in psychotherapy. In G.R. Vandenbos (Ed.), *Psychotherapy: practice, research, policy,* (pp.103-162), Beverly Hills, CA: Sage.

Zigmond, A.S. & Snaith, R.P. (1983). The Hospital Anxiety and Depression Scale. *Acta Psychiatr. Scand., 67,* 361-370